Curing Crohn's

How A Closet Food Addict Healed Her IBD

Cassidy Gundersen

This book contains the opinions, religious beliefs, and ideas of the author. Although there is no cure for Crohn's disease, the word 'cure' in the title is used to describe the author's own personal health journey in a way that a majority of people may understand. This book is only intended to provide helpful, general information on the subjects it addresses. It does not in any way represent a substitute for the advice of the reader's own physician or other medical professionals based on the reader's own individual conditions, symptoms, or concerns. If the reader needs personal medical, health, or dietary assistance or advice, the reader should consult a competent physician or other qualified health care professional. The author and publisher specifically disclaim all responsibility for injury, damage, or loss that the reader may incur as a direct or indirect consequence of following any directions or suggestions given in this book.

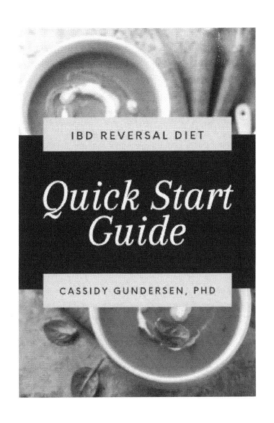

IBD REVERSAL DIET

Quick Start Guide

CASSIDY GUNDERSEN, PHD

Get the FREE Quick Start Guide!

https://reverseibd.com/quick-start

To the two men who made me whole–my husband Jordan, and my Savior Jesus Christ.

With their aid, I have found healing.

Introduction

An estimated 700 million people across the world have one or more autoimmune diseases, and that number is on the rise.[1] Since there are over 100 known autoimmune diseases, the symptoms vary widely. Such illnesses range from affecting the thyroid, to the bones, to the GI tract, to the brain. You name it and autoimmune disease can affect it. Each person afflicted with an autoimmune condition is suffering not only physically, but spiritually, mentally, and even financially. Healthcare costs are five times higher for someone with a chronic disease compared to someone without.[2] It is no wonder that these diseases are the number one cause of bankruptcy in the United States.[3]

Just one of these diseases, inflammatory bowel disease (IBD), accounts for over 3 million cases in the United States as of 2015.[4] An additional 12 percent, over 37 million Americans, are subject to irritable bowel syndrome (IBS).[5] With over 40 million Americans suffering from these digestive woes, one would think that further strides and advances would have been made in finding a cure. At least that's what I thought when I was diagnosed in 2013. I asked each new specialist and doctor I met with if there was hope for me to be cured. Each assured me there was no cure, but if I played my cards right, I might be able to manage it with medication. When I discovered that there were dozens of peer-reviewed studies that indicated that 100 percent remission rate was not only possible but easily achieved with diet and lifestyle changes, I was floored! I spent hours and hours combing through the data and made a plan for myself.

After careful and methodical planning, I sprung into action. My success caught wind with many of my friends and family, and before I knew it, people started looking to me as an IBD and IBS expert. As I started to educate people with nearly every digestive disorder in the book, I saw the same principles yield incredible results, and I knew I had to reach a wider audience.

Since that time, I have been doing all I can to get the message out there! This was one of the main reasons why I wrote this book. Putting your full weight behind a message isn't all fun and games, however. I have faced my fair share of pushback, but the principles contained in this book are tried and true. I have watched seemingly miraculous healing occur with many people, some of whom you will read about in the book, as they forsook everything they thought they knew about health and tried this new way.

What we will discuss in this book is radical, not because it is revolutionary, but because it is vastly different from what has been taught in medical schools and in the offices of Gastroenterologists. This should come as no surprise since less than 4 percent of Gastroenterologists in the United States use nutritional therapy as a primary form of treatment.[6] Nevertheless, these things are true not only because I have seen them work, but because of the hundreds of peer reviewed studies that back them up.

This book is also radical because it shows a route toward complete healing, not just management. Most other approaches focus on ways to barely skirt around a flare up, or how to feel good on medication. However, each one of my clients (and myself) has eventually come to a point where medication is not only useless but a hindrance in their IBD or IBS journey. Though work will have to be done and sacrifices made to ensure you stay healthy, there is no need to be worried about a flare-up or medical emergency when you are eating the right way.

In this book, you will hear my story of disaster and subsequent change and healing. After this, I will lay out a 4-step plan for you to get your life back. This will include important steps and specific things to focus on and to avoid. This is where you will get a look at my game plan. I have also compiled a few stories from some of my coaching clients to encourage you and help you feel hope for the future. Finally, we'll tackle some hard questions in the FAQs chapter.

This is in no way a conclusive look at healing IBD and autoimmune disease, and there are a number of considerations for each individual. However, these principles can help you get on the right track. In some cases, small changes will make a big difference; healing can often be felt shortly after applying these principles. Yet, other cases take a few months of maneuvering and fine-tuning. Whatever your case, know that you are not alone; numerous others have taken the same route and have all found healing.

It is important to note that I am not a medical doctor. Nothing that I write in this book should be construed as medical advice. There is currently no known medical "cure" for Crohn's disease or other forms of IBD. In this book, I use the word "cure" to denote 100 percent remission. In my own coaching practice, I do not prescribe or treat any kind of disease, I simply teach people the correct principles, and let them choose and implement for themselves. This is because I believe that the responsibility for health lies with the individual–not an outside party such as a doctor, surgeon, or any other kind of practitioner. Therefore, I encourage each person to evaluate and research the information in this book regarding disease and nutrition to make informed decisions about his or her own health. I can't make any guarantees regarding your health and the information in this book. However, I can probably guarantee that you have not heard a story quite like the one you're about to read.

Chapter One

How I Got Sick

"And the winner of Miss Idaho 2012 is ... Cassidy Bronson." It took me a few seconds to realize that the announcer was talking about me! I stepped up in disbelief as they crowned me and put my new sash on. I kept asking myself, "Is this real life?" I was so elated, I could barely think. I had been competing in and winning pageants for many years, but this one was top on my list. After press interviews, a series of pictures, and an acceptance speech, it was time for the pageant after-party–the best part. After accepting my awards for physical fitness, I indulged in an entire pizza by myself. By this time in my life, I had learned that people would often question me if they saw me eating all of that food at one time. I made sure I only grabbed a slice at a time and walked around to ensure I was not with the same people while I ate. Then I headed over for a slice of cake. Okay, two slices of cake. Alright, maybe it was more like six or seven pieces. Even though I was stuffed, I had yet to have my customary post-pageant cookie dough. After each pageant I did (starting at age 13), I would treat myself to an entire roll of packaged cookie dough. I ended my night with a crown on my head and a lot of food in my stomach. What no one else would have guessed is that I had likely eaten more than 4000 calories of food that evening, not including the cookies, brownies, and chocolates I had stuffed my face with backstage before the pageant. If you were to ask me more about my memories from winning Miss Idaho, I couldn't tell you many specifics from the event itself, but I can describe the food I ate in very fine detail. This is also true for many major events in my life. At the time, I didn't know any different. I had no inkling that this kind of behavior was not only unhealthy, but a recipe for disaster. What I would later learn was that despite looking beautiful on the outside, I was a wreck on the inside. My life was a façade; it was fake, much like the "food" I was eating. What I didn't realize was that I was addicted to these products–they were my drug of choice.

From a very young age, food has always been a big part of my life. It might be hard to believe, but my first word as a baby was "taco." Home videos show me constantly asking for and raving about various chocolaty treats and sugar-filled baked goods. The essence of my childhood is best captured in an experience I had as a toddler. When I was around 18 months old, I was in the kitchen baking cookies with my mom when she left for a moment to answer the door or go to the bathroom. When she came back, I was gone along with the large bowl of cookie dough. After searching for a few minutes, my mom found me on the stairs covered in cookie dough. Somehow I had managed to eat almost an entire bowl of cookie dough in one sitting, and I wasn't even two years old! Although this sounds cute and somewhat silly, this experience would mark the beginning of my relationship with food for the rest of my life—a relationship that would eventually lead me to a diagnosis of Crohn's disease. What many people don't realize is that Crohn's disease, inflammatory bowel disease (IBD), and irritable bowel syndrome (IBS) don't typically just come on suddenly. They usually form over many years due to a combination of poor nutrition, stress, and many other factors. Of course, everyone has a different experience, but I feel that my story is particularly unique. Hopefully, through the telling of my story, you will be able to see that if I was able to find hope and healing, there can be hope and healing for you as well.

Before we get too far into my story, I feel that it is appropriate to level with you. The title of the book is called Curing Crohn's. However, the medical community will tell you that there is no cure for

Crohn's disease or IBD, and they are right. There is no drug or treatment that will cure Crohn's disease. Cure, in fact, is a funny word that is ill-defined and no longer used in the typical health lexicon. Interestingly enough, only medical doctors can treat, prescribe, and cure when it comes to disease, and even then, most would avoid using the word "cure" to avoid liability and lawsuits in their practices. The most acceptable word to use regarding IBD is "remission." But what is the difference between "100 percent remission," "heal," "reverse," and "cure?" When one no longer experiences the symptoms of a disease (and doctors can no longer find evidence of its existence in the body), does it really matter what word you use to describe the wonderful relief? In my mind, these are synonymous, but you might disagree. I should note, however, that because I am not a medical doctor, I am not offering a "cure" for Crohn's disease. This is a story about when I hit rock bottom and vowed that I would find a cure for myself. Your cure might look different than mine did, but there are principles that work for everyone. This is what I want to tell you about–the principles that helped me and many others to reverse their health challenges, IBD or otherwise. This book is about how I took these principles, changed my food choices, and went from a fake, chronically ill lifestyle to one that is real, raw, and healthy.

As a child born in the 1990s, my favorite toy was the "Easy Bake Oven." I would bake treats as often as I could, even when we didn't have the special "Easy Bake Oven" ingredients. This led me to create my own recipes for cookies and cakes and desserts of all kinds. Going grocery shopping with my mom was always a delight because I could influence what we would be eating and what treats we would be making. At this young age, I often dreamed of combining my love of performing and my love of food into the ultimate job: a Miss America grocery bagger. I dreamed of wearing a crown and high heels to work each day to bag the groceries of local shoppers—a dream I would one day live out.

By age seven, I had fallen in love with singing. I sang every chance I could get, usually winning many competitions. Each time I was in a competition, my mom would reward me by treating me to ice cream or donuts. My mom and many other people could bribe me to do nearly anything if there was a promise of donuts at the end. Donuts were my kryptonite. Another one of my kryptonite foods was bacon. I would set off the fire alarm nearly once a week trying to cook bacon.

When I was eight years old, I won the first of many pageants. After winning, my mom asked what I wanted to do to celebrate. I immediately expressed my desire to order asphalt pie and wings at Wingers. So with the newly-earned crown on my head, I went in and stuffed my face. Later that year, I attended my first summer camp. Because I thought the water tasted disgusting, I drank only soda for the entire week of the camp.

Throughout my tween years I came up with a new dream: having my very own cooking show like Martha Stewart. I would often line the kitchen table with stuffed animals or force my siblings to watch as I made all kinds of baked goods and strange concoctions as if I had my own TV show. I would pre-measure everything out and explain each ingredient. Every single treat had a solid base of butter, sugar, and white flour while the rest was up to my imagination. When I wasn't cooking, you could find me performing my heart out on stage. I traveled around the world performing on various cruise lines, at Disney World, in Europe, and I was even a Radio Disney spokesperson. A lot of stress and a busy schedule made me the prime candidate for a serious lifestyle disease.

By age 13, most of my life was focused around food. I say food but a more appropriate term is junk food. I lived for junk food. I would earn quarters and search for money around the house so that instead of buying a proper middle school lunch, I could buy a caffeinated drink and creme-filled chocolate pastries. When my mom started buying food for us to make home lunches, my meals changed to a soda, a bag of chips, a store-bought cookie or treat (of which I would often sneak two or three), and a sandwich. The only kind of sandwich I would eat was on white bread, with peanut butter and marshmallow fluff. No one could have ever guessed I ate like this, however, because I still hadn't broken 90 lbs., and I towered over most of my peers at 5' 8".

At this time, I was cast in my dream role as Eponine in the Broadway hit musical Les Miserables. I also won the title of Miss Teen Idaho–the youngest teen in Idaho's history to win that pageant. It was a shock to everyone, including me! You probably wouldn't believe that while everyone was eating salad backstage in preparation for the pageant, I was stuffing my face with pizza, but it's true. Nothing was going to stop me from eating what I wanted. I was excited but had little idea of the pressures that awaited such a triumph. As I met with the pageant directors the day after winning, we began making preparations for intense vocal lessons, a workout regimen, spray tans, and travel plans for my two-week trip to Orlando for the national Miss Teen America pageant. It hit me that my life was about to be much busier and more stressful than ever before.

I spent very little time in school that year and instead spent a great deal of time on the road singing and speaking to audiences across the country. Sounds like a dream for such a young girl to accomplish so much, doesn't it? But it didn't come without a cost. I had all the praise of the world, but I wasn't happy. My addiction to food grew even deeper and my outward health finally took an inevitable turn for the worse.

I thought my trip to the national Miss Teen America pageant would be no different from the luxurious and seemingly care-free life I had been living, but I was wrong. As I arrived alone in Orlando for my two weeks of pageanting, I became very ill. I found myself in extreme pain and couldn't get out of bed for an entire day. I slept for nearly 24 hours and woke only to go to the bathroom, which was excruciating. At the time I didn't realize it, but these were the beginning signs that my digestion and body were deteriorating. By the second day of intense stomach pains, the directors advised that I be taken to a nearby emergency room. So, I was taken to the ER where I was treated with all kinds of medications and tests and sent back on my way 12 hours later. I arrived back at the hotel room drowsy and still in pain. With no answers as to what was happening, I continued the medications and pressed on through the long two weeks at the pageant.

My First Kidney Stone

I came home from the experience and felt like I had recovered fairly well. However, during a trip to Arizona later that year, everything changed. When I traveled, I often lived on Pop Tarts, Doritos, packaged cookies, and marshmallows. This trip was no different. On our way back home, I began feeling extreme side pain which persisted for nearly 24 hours. At first, I thought I had sore muscles, but as the pain progressed, I thought perhaps it was a pinched nerve. I stretched, had some ibuprofen, and tried to sleep it off. I remember feeling sick and unable to go to the bathroom or eat, but I chalked it up to traveling inconveniences and tried to press forward.

By the next morning, I knew I was dealing with something far worse than a pinched nerve. I was in so much pain that the only thing I could do was lie in the fetal position and cry. The pain was so unbearable that I began throwing up profusely, still unable to voluntarily move myself. I knew something was terribly wrong. I felt like I was going to die, and it was unimaginable to me that the human body could endure such intense pain. The pain that started in my back radiated through my entire side and enveloped the right half of my body. I remember praying so earnestly, begging God to "please let this pass or let me pass." Little did I know, the only thing that really needed to pass was a large kidney stone stuck in my urinary tract.

I had no idea at the time, but this first kidney stone at the young age of 13 would mark the beginning of a lifelong struggle with kidney stones, having multiple kidney stone attacks each year. Though my first attack was one that I would vividly remember for the rest of my life, more painful episodes were soon to follow. I would often find myself panicking each time my side began to ache or my urine was changed in any way. I would immediately reach for my prescribed oxycodone to numb the pain before it worsened to any degree. This vigilance, however, was always to no avail. Regardless of which medications I took, how much counter pressure, heat, or ice was applied, the pain wouldn't subside.

I was given some vague instructions by the doctor to not take calcium supplements, but other than that I was in the dark as to what was causing my issues. I was also not given any hope that I would ever be able to live without fear of the next attack. With no direction from the doctor and virtually no knowledge of health and nutrition myself, I went on with my eating habits feeling certain that there was no way they could be linked to my health problems.

At this point in my story, there is something you should know about me when it comes to pain: I was as tough as they come. I rarely cried when in pain, but each time I had a kidney stone, I couldn't contain the tears. Begging for help and for release, I would go through a typical attack that would last around 24 hours of intense pain, and then I would sleep for the next 24 hours. I figured out what worked for me, and I hunkered down each time a new kidney stone would make its way through my little body.

Fifty years ago, hearing that a young child suffered from chronic kidney stones would have been shocking to most people. Though kidney stones are still a fairly rare occurrence in children these days, the number of children affected has risen significantly. The largest contributor to this problem, I believe, is diet. Kids now live on sodium and sugar-filled products that provide little nutritional value. Fast food, frozen meals, lunch meats, chips, candy, soft drinks–all of these things can lead to the development of kidney stones, especially when you have inflamed bowels and digestive problems like I did.[7]

Childhood Diet

You might be wondering, "how are kidney stones related to IBD?" You might think that they are not at all related, but the body is a complete organism. When something is wrong, the body will send out signals and warnings trying to get our attention. But oftentimes we fail to recognize that these warnings indicate much larger trouble in the body, so we begin to work on the effect, not the root cause of the problem. Most of the diseases we see today appear not because the body is breaking down, but because the body has not been properly fed. Most disease actually starts in the bowels. When I discovered this, it became obvious that it wasn't just my love of sweets and junk food that caused my problems, it was pretty much everything I ate while growing up. As a child, I was an extremely picky eater. Many are surprised to learn that I have no memories of trying a pear, date, fig, mango, coconut, avocado, sweet potato, or many other items until my mid-twenties after I was married. I remember the first time I had a mango, thinking I had discovered an incredible new fringe food that no one else knew about. After I began telling people how incredible they were, I quickly realized that everyone else knew all about mangoes long before I had even heard of them.

Our family didn't often go out to eat, but when I would accompany my mom for business meetings, she would usually go to McDonald's or, my personal favorite, Arby's. I have many memories of my mom ordering five roast beef sandwiches in the "5 for $5" deals at Arby's and I would eat all five sandwiches. When we would go on trips, I would save my money to order a burger, fries, and a large shake at In-N-Out or Jack-In-The-Box. My favorite vacations were the cruises we went on because they had all-you-can-eat desserts and a midnight chocolate buffet, which surely accounted for most of my calorie intake on those trips.

Like many other homes in the early 2000s, we were allowed to have unlimited amounts of three products (not foods) growing up: ramen, macaroni and cheese, and bulk sugar cereals. When we were hungry, we were allowed to eat those foods and nothing else. Consequently, those items ended up comprising a large portion of my diet at home. Beyond those things, we had a lot of casseroles and traditional southern dishes because my mother grew up in the deep south. Cream cheese chicken, steak stroganoff, cheesy potato soup, pot roast, chicken and biscuits, and Krusteaz pancakes made up most of my childhood family dinners. If there was ever a side salad or canned fruit cocktail, I would always avoid those items like the plague.

My mom was an incredible baker, and she would make desserts several times each week. I would often come home from school to the smell of fresh baked cookies waiting on the counter. Many evenings after my younger siblings would go to sleep, my dad and I would share a large bowl of ice cream topped with peanut butter and occasionally chocolate fudge. I do not have a memory of a single day from my childhood going without some kind of treat or candy. When I was feeling "healthy" I would eat an off-brand version of Lucky Charms, Fruit Loops, or Frosted Flakes. I would also opt for eating a block of cheese or processed deli meats.

The biggest problem with all of these "foods" I ate every single day is that hardly any of them were actually real foods that came from the ground! My parents, like almost every American, were products of a failed nutrition education program in the United States which taught that all food is created equal. My parents did what they thought was healthy after being educated by the food industry interests. Like so many others, they were taught to embrace hormone-rich dairy products. We were told that canned was just as good as fresh. We were taught that processed food was fine, especially if it was "low fat." I credit the corporate nutrition establishment for our family's poor eating habits, as with the habits of millions of others as well.

Once a Month

It seems that these days the rage is "gut health." In order to be healthy, they say, you have to have a healthy gut. This is a very true sentiment, as most diseases start in the bowels. But what most people don't realize is that good gut health is determined by how well your bowels are moving. When I was young, they simply weren't. A story from when I was a newlywed best illustrates my understanding of bowel movements and their importance for most of my life.

In 2015, I had met and married the love of my life. We had a beautiful outdoor wedding reception in mid-

August. After our reception, we spent a week on a honeymoon before we moved to Washington DC. It was a whirlwind, and I was exhausted from the wedding and the events surrounding it.The first few weeks of marriage were a blur, but one morning after we had been married for about a month, my husband, Jordan, was in the bathroom for his usual morning bowel movement. This was beginning to be annoying to me since it seemed to take up such a large part of each morning. As I was getting ready in the bedroom, I asked through the door, "Why do you poop so much? It can't be good to go to the bathroom every single day."

Jordan laughed and quickly responded, "You're supposed to have a bowel movement every day, but I don't think I've ever seen you poop."

I laughed back at him and said, "No you're not! That's *way* too often. I go once a month."

He gasped in utter shock: "Once a month?!"

I was sure I was right, but I was also slightly embarrassed, so we quickly turned to Google to settle the debate. I was absolutely amazed to discover that doctors recommended that people have a bowel movement at least once a day on average. I had never heard such a thing before in my entire life.

For as long as I could remember, I had had a single bowel movement each month, many times accompanying my period. That's right, I pooped about twelve times a year! Doctors had often asked if I was "regular," but how was I supposed to know what that meant? I didn't have anyone to ask since such things weren't proper to talk about in my home. So I always just responded in the affirmative. For years, I had been chronically constipated, and I had no idea.

Later, I would learn that even just a single bowel movement in a day was a sign of constipation, and that a healthy person should excrete these toxins at least three to four times a day. We will discuss this in a later chapter, but suffice it to say I have yet to meet a single person who has had as few bowel movements as I did.

Go, Go, Go

My poor eating habits, as you can guess, continued when I became a teenager. I won the title of Miss Teen Idaho under other pageant organizations two additional times, and with this came a whole host of additional problems. In news interviews, appearances around the United States, performing for all kinds of events, and competing at nationals, I may have been a poster child of beauty on the outside, but my insides were certainly not beautiful. As my life got busier, my diet got worse. When we were busy or traveling, I would rely more on fast, pre-prepared, and processed foods.

Although my diet consisted mainly of chemicals and toxins, for some odd reason I refused to drink impure water. I thought tap water was gross, so I wouldn't drink it unless it had been purified. That often meant that while I was on the road or away from home I would either be severely dehydrated from a lack of water, or that I would live exclusively on soda or juice.

When I was 15 years old I landed a leading role in a play that required me to move to St. George, Utah alone for the summer. Being the youngest in the cast and without a car, I was beholden to my older friends for a ride to the grocery store, but that was no issue for me. That summer I was powered by cookies, crackers, frozen pastries, hot pockets, chicken nuggets, and a sugar-filled drink that was intended to resemble peach juice. Frequent shopping trips were clearly not necessary since the actual expiration dates of those items would have been years later. That summer I began experiencing extreme fatigue and stomach cramping which would only worsen as the years went on.

It's no wonder that at 16 years old, I had debilitating PMS symptoms each time my period would come, which was sporadically every few months. My cramps would be horrible and I could do nothing but lie in bed for the first two days of my period. At one point we thought that I might have endometriosis or PCOS, though this was never confirmed.

Through all of these experiences, I never gained the weight that would be expected for such an avid and unhealthy eater. I didn't break 100 lbs. until I was in college. I even modeled for a number of companies throughout my teenage years. Perhaps the greatest achievement from these years (and the years to come) was fooling so many people that I was very healthy. But the cracks in this façade were starting to show, and I began to worry that people would find out my secret. I was an absolute food addict. I was miserable inside and out, but no one would have ever known. The greatest deception, however, was yet to come.

Miss Idaho and American Idol

As I entered my twenties, my already busy and hectic life grew even crazier. At the beginning of the year, I decided to re-enter the pageant world. In the spring of 2012, I won the Miss Idaho pageant. This brought even more stress and health problems, exacerbating my pre-existing conditions of kidney stones, PMS complications, and chronic fatigue. Ironically enough, I won the health and fitness competition of the pageant! By every outward standard, this was true. Of course, it also helped that despite my poor inward health, I could hop on a bike a few days before a pageant and shed excess body fat. However, I was the only one who knew this couldn't be more laughable, because by this point, I was often missing work and school due to health problems. I knew how to say all the right things and wear all the right clothes to elevate myself and hide my worsening health.

Perhaps the greatest of all the ironies is that the platform I advocated and won on was improving women's health. I talked about access to clean water and its importance, as well as nutritional deficiencies of mothers around the world, failing to realize that my own nutritional deficiencies would soon nearly kill me. My greatest memory of winning the title was, of course, the epic after-party! Fancy desserts and sparkling apple cider filled me to the brim, and I slept in late the next morning. Despite never having touched alcohol in my life, I seemed to experience "food hangovers" quite often. I would binge eat and spend the next day lying in bed trying to recover. Being Miss Idaho added a whole new element to this lifestyle.

When I became Miss Idaho, my mom set up an opportunity for me to go to the grocery store. It was there that I fulfilled my childhood dream and became the Miss Idaho grocery bagger in my crown, sash, and high heels. I loved the attention and praise that this accomplishment brought me, but there was something missing. My life seemed to be like a seesaw with very high highs and very low lows, especially when it came to my health.

Even though I could hide the problem of my worsening health, I couldn't hide the poor habits. I was Miss Idaho, and everyone was more interested in my title and fame. They couldn't care less about what I ate for breakfast. Each time I would go on a date with a boy, he would joke about how horribly I ate and still seemed so skinny. One boy keenly observed, "You're like a junk food barbie." My suitors knew that the way to my heart was through my stomach. Boys would often surprise me with homemade pies, juicy burgers, or store-bought treats.

I always felt ill, but because I didn't know any different, I had convinced myself that my problems were simply because I wasn't working hard enough. The logical solution was to work harder. I figured that the only reason other people didn't sleep as much as I did was because I was lazy. With that pretense, I added to my already full plate by joining the Model United Nations team at Brigham Young University. I missed many practices due to kidney stones and other health problems, but ultimately earned a spot on the top competitive team and was selected to compete in New York at the United Nations tournament. At that tournament, my team won the highest award, and my partner and I were recognized as a top partnership from teams competing from around the world. Just like all of my previous experiences though, that trip was characterized by which restaurants we ate at and how many famous New York cheesecakes we could eat in one sitting. It should have come as no surprise to me that I had an intense migraine and accompanying stomach pain that almost landed me in the ER while there.

It was a few months after this trip to New York that I traveled to Chicago for the big pageant with all the contestants from around America. When we flew into town, the first thing I did was find the nearest Chicago deep dish pizza parlor and indulge in an entire pizza by myself. Like the others that came before, this trip would also land me in the hospital. In fact, each one of my pageant experiences would end up with me incredibly sick and either at the hospital or stuck in bed. The high stress associated with these competitions overworked my already fatigued nervous system. Consequently, I would end up an emotional wreck and would resort to binge eating. I would hide these feelings with every food you can imagine–except healthy ones, of course. The upscale hotel we stayed at for the competition offered free fresh baked chocolate chip cookies in the lounge every day. I managed to sneak eight to ten cookies per day from the lounge and eat them between rehearsals, interviews and preparations. Additionally, I sent my mom to the grocery store to ensure that I had raw cookie dough on hand to eat each night when I came home–you know, the ritual. The greatest contrast between me and the other contestants was that while they were eating salad, I was often eating second and third helpings of hearty meals.

A pageant is much more work than most people realize. It's not about pounding on the makeup and wearing a pretty dress, although that is definitely a part of it. It is usually one to two weeks of interviews, media appearances, dress rehearsals, service projects, banquets, charity auctions, and more. At these events each day is performance, and though you might be on stage for just a few hours, there is a great amount of stress all day every day. It's no wonder I was sick at every pageant! Being "on" all day every day takes its toll, and mine manifested itself in illness.

In addition to everything already on my plate I decided to throw caution to the wind and audition for American Idol. Much to my surprise, I kept getting selected to continue round after round. Soon I found myself in LA competing on the weekends for the largest singing competition in America. Each time I traveled to LA, I ate. . .well, I'm sure you can guess what my eating habits looked like: junk, burgers, desserts, and soda.

As the competition grew more intense, so did my anxiety and health problems. During the season that I competed, I was brushing shoulders with Nikki Minaj, Mariah Carey, Keith Urban, and others. On one occasion the producers were interviewing me about my lifelong crush on Keith Urban and my joy at being able to meet him, while, unbeknownst to me, he was standing behind me the whole time and proceeded to say, "I love you too darling." Embarrassed but giddy, I knew I would never forget that moment. I primped and prepared, and the cameras were always watching. American Idol behind the scenes is nothing like you would expect. It's a lot of waiting, very little actual drama, and a scripted outcome. Regardless, with all the other things I had on my plate, my capacity for dealing with stress was diminishing quickly, and my body was giving out.

After one particularly difficult week with school, a quick trip to LA, and then back up to Idaho for some Miss Idaho appearances, my body crashed. Hard. I couldn't get out of bed for more than 36 hours. My memories of that week are shoddy, but it was bad enough that I missed every single one of my semester finals and barely ate a single thing the whole week. My whole world came crashing down on me, and at moments I was sure I must have cancer or some other terminal illness. My symptoms were across the board and even doctors didn't know what to tell me. My entire life had built up to this and every single cake, soda, and dessert snack was attacking me all at once. I cried out to God, "Is this it? Am I going to die? How is it possible to be in so much pain?" Little did I know, I would survive this incident, but the worst was yet to come. Soon, I would receive my gut-wrenching diagnosis.

Chapter Two

The Crohn's Diagnosis

Gaining Weight

After I recovered from my terrible incident, I moved home to Idaho before deciding to leave my current lifestyle behind and become a missionary for my church. After completing the necessary application, I was assigned to go to Winnipeg, Canada for 18 months. I wouldn't have access to social media or my own phone and I would get to call home twice a year on Mother's Day and Christmas–a stark contrast to the life I had been living. The days would be long and difficult, but I was craving a break from my hectic life. Though the glamour and glitz were exciting, I yearned for something real and authentic. I hoped that I would find this in Canada.

While living in Canada, my health continued to drastically decline. The headaches were getting more frequent, and I began experiencing intense stomach pains as well. One day I landed myself in the ER after a great deal of pain and numbness in my body. Within two months of this time, I had gained nearly 60 lbs! This was a difficult reality for someone who had spent the previous year being Miss Idaho. Despite my severe food addiction, I had been blessed with a lightning fast metabolism and good genes. Throughout my entire life I had been known for my skinny body and good looks. It was a very difficult realization that all of that was gone. As if my health problems weren't bad enough, I also lost a lot of confidence that came from my slim figure.

One of the families I interacted with frequently were immigrants from the Philippines. They were a kind and loving family, but they pulled no punches and were brutally honest. They surely noticed my rapid weight gain, because on one occasion while teaching in their home, the teenage boy said, "Wow, Sister Bronson, you have gotten really fat!" He felt bad about saying this and later showed up at our door with a bag of candy as an apology. But he wasn't wrong. I had put on so much weight, I didn't know what to do. My clothes no longer fit, my hair was beginning to fall out, and I was dealing with much larger health concerns than just my weight.

The Crohn's Diagnosis

After an experience I had with a deer carcass in the home of a member of our church, I couldn't bring myself to eat meat anymore and immediately went vegetarian. Despite foregoing one of the biggest contributing foods to IBD, my issues didn't improve. After going vegetarian, I increased my eggs, dairy, and bread intake. Though I began to make a conscious effort for the first time in my life to eat a bit healthier, very few fruits and vegetables sounded appetizing to me. I began to make scrambled eggs and toast each morning for breakfast –sometimes I would gag down a banana with it, but rarely could I make it through the whole thing. I tried hard during this phase to not drink any soda, though occasionally I would indulge. Still, these were the least of my problems. My cupboard was still constantly lined with candy bars and packaged pastries.

It was around this time that I became even more concerned about my health. I recounted in my journal, "I feel like I'm going to die!" I noticed that during my occasional bowel movements, there would be copious amounts of blood. I also had severe pain, which I would later learn was caused by hemorrhoids. This was accompanied by bouts of extreme sickness and nausea. Despite all of this, I stopped myself from saying anything for fear of being sent home from my mission. It wasn't until I started noticing blood in my saliva every time I brushed my teeth, that I became worried and decided it was time to get help.

During a trip I took training other missionaries, my pain got to a point that I couldn't handle anymore, and we went to the ER again, only to wait all day. Once I was finally able to get in and get examined, the doctor informed me that they believed I had Crohn's disease. I had no idea what that was or what it entailed. I was in complete shock, and I didn't know what to ask other than, what can I do about it? He said that there was nothing I could do but take the pills–the typical answer from almost all doctors. He prescribed me some medications and told me to schedule a visit with a gastroenterologist. I was unable to set up an appointment with the gastroenterologist for several weeks but waited patiently for the day I would get more information. In the meantime, the pain was almost unbearable, and I had convinced myself the doctor was wrong. I visited another ER in a different city in hopes of getting a different diagnosis and additional help. Unfortunately, this doctor and his tests determined the same thing. During the first diagnosis I was in denial and never fully accepted it. However, when the second doctor confirmed what the first had said, I was a wreck. I was so emotional and felt so hopeless.

Before this point, I had never considered myself to have digestive problems. Looking back, however, I wonder how the thought had never crossed my mind.

Though many with IBD have severe diarrhea, I was one of the minority who had quite the opposite battle. For years, I had infrequent bowel movements, but over the past few years the pain had grown exponentially. I was bloated, gassy, and had extremely painful bowel movements that were always accompanied by blood. My stomach would often make loud and embarrassing noises, and I had been diagnosed with a number of stomach ulcers throughout my life. All of this cumulatively should have given me plenty of red flags, but I guess it wasn't enough. The diagnosis of Crohn's disease came as a complete shock. The confident girl who had captivated audiences in a designer gown just a year before was now overweight, sick, and falling apart.

I had big plans and dreams, and yet I could barely make it through the day. I loathed medication. Even when I began taking it, I didn't notice any improvement in my symptoms. In fact, I became more tired and lethargic than ever before. If there was a lull in a conversation, I would fall asleep. I became angry and wondered how I could endure this pain for the rest of my life.

When I was finally able to meet with the gastroenterologist, I had accepted my diagnosis. The anger was gone, but I still felt completely hopeless. By this point, I was willing to do anything that might give me relief. At the appointment, I asked as many questions as I could. I was even willing to change my diet! To my dismay, he informed me that foods didn't cause flares and that I was free to eat whatever I wanted, which I continued to do. He did, however, tell me that I needed to eat a liquid diet for one week at the start of my medication and that would possibly help relieve symptoms.

Trying to Get Healthy

During my one-week liquid diet, I worked hard to only drink juice and eat soup. It was incredibly hard for me to give up all of my favorite foods and have enough self-control to just have liquids. On multiple occasions I would sneak solid foods while my companion was in the other room. I knew that the doctor had ordered me to eat liquids, but I couldn't follow through. This experience did, however, convince me to begin looking for ways to improve my health.

At this point in my mission, I was living in Saskatchewan and was lucky enough to be in an area of very health-conscious people. Many of the people we were teaching and many members of the church in that area were very healthy. I knew that I needed to make changes in order to get better, but I didn't know what those changes would be. I began by asking everyone I knew. It was there that I was introduced to edamame beans, kombucha, fermentation, juicing, sprouting, and much more for the first time in my life. Previous to this, I had never heard of or considered these things. I would spend hours talking to these health gurus and figuring out what they did and why.

The biggest shift that I made during this time was to stop buying all of my sugary treats and go-to snacks. I knew that those things were not good for me, and I made a concerted effort to avoid them. I knew that I needed something else, so I filled the void with chocolate covered almonds. This was perhaps the healthiest treat I had ever had in my whole life. I enjoyed them and bought several pounds each week.

I also began taking wheatgrass, as I heard that it helped with inflammation and stomach problems. While it tasted disgusting, I always had so much energy afterwards. Every time I could get my hands on some kind of juice, herb, supplement or anything else I thought might be healthy, I jumped at the opportunity. Though I knew very little about health, I noticed differences when I used these healthy things that others recommended. I began to wonder if perhaps these foods and herbs could heal me in time. I wanted to learn as much as I could about nutrition from these healthy people.

During the closing weeks of my 18-month mission, I was convinced that I had no other options than to be sick my whole life. Just a few years previous, I had been a revered beauty queen, traveling the nation and showing off my confidence on stage in heels and sparkles. Now I was a sickly, overweight, and exhausted woman with no confidence and little hope for my future. Many people who I had interacted with during these difficult times would probably be shocked to learn that I was as sick as I was, physically and mentally. I forced myself up out of bed each morning, despite every inch of my body telling me not to. I worked as hard as I could and worked my body into the ground.

Old Habits Die Hard

As my mission came to a close, I was relieved to go home and work on getting myself better. When I arrived home, I tried my hardest to keep up the good eating habits that I had developed near the end of my mission. I was worried about how I would be able to accomplish this in a new environment and with a new lifestyle. Unfortunately, it only took days before I fell back into old habits.

When we arrived home, a family friend had brought over a basket to welcome me back, and I ate every chocolate covered pretzel from the basket that first night. I hoped that being home in Idaho would somehow make my growing list of conditions disappear so that I could get back to a "normal" life. But that just didn't seem to be in the cards for me. I found myself sleeping for extremely long periods, and I struggled to find a job that would accommodate my continued health problems.

What I lacked in health and energy, however, I made up for in suitors. When I came home, I was welcomed by a lot of young men eager to take me on a date. It was both flattering and stressful, particularly because in the Mormon culture people tend to get married young. Once again, I turned to food to numb my emotions. But I also used this to my advantage. I would always arrange for my dates to be at a restaurant or to have food somehow involved. The boys I dated quickly picked up on my love of food, and would often show up with my favorite tempura vegetables, ginger ale, oreo cakesters, or granola. To their credit, they knew the way to my heart.

"Food Won't Affect Your Digestion"

Though I was more health conscious than ever before, I still often snuck desserts and treats. And by often I mean at least once a day. There was not a day that would go by that I wouldn't resort to some kind of chocolate or sugary treat. When things were stressful, my eating habits became worse. I often felt guilty because at the end of my mission I had learned that food was important. However, I still had no idea to what degree I would be impacted by my food choices.

After being home for a short period of time, I began seeing more specialized doctors who I thought might be able to give me more answers. My symptoms were getting worse and I began to experience additional concerning symptoms. I wanted answers, and I was getting to the point where I was willing to try whatever it took to get better.

On one occasion, I was meeting with a gastroenterologist in Idaho, and he was telling me about the results of my latest blood work. He told me that I was deficient in nearly every category. We talked through the vitamins and pills he suggested as well as additional testing that would be needed. I told him that I wasn't as much concerned about all the other problems and that I just wanted my Crohn's disease to get better. I asked what I needed to do to get better. I said, "Tell me what foods to avoid, what foods to focus on, what to eat and not eat–I'll do it! Just tell me what's best." His response changed the course of my life forever.

In that pivotal moment looking for answers to my health challenges, he looked me square in the eyes and said, "Food won't affect your digestion. It doesn't matter what you eat. Just focus on the medication, and we will go from there." Let me repeat that: he said food does not affect digestion, implying that all foods are created equal and it doesn't matter what you eat! I think my jaw dropped to the floor when he said those words. I didn't know much about health or nutrition, but something told me that wasn't true. Funny enough, I had graduated from high school early and managed to avoid taking the required health class. But again, there was a part of me that thought, "I may not know anything about health, and I'm by no means a doctor, but it makes absolutely no sense for me to have severe stomach and digestive pains that are not associated in any way to the foods I eat."

I didn't know it at the time, but I would later learn that less than 4% of American gastroenterologists use nutrition and lifestyle as a primary form of treatment.[8] This is a travesty because, as we will discuss later, nutrition is the biggest contributor to Crohn's disease and to healing it. The problem is simply that doctors don't learn this in medical school. If they come across any of the hundreds of peer-reviewed studies on the impacts of diet on IBD and IBS, it is generally on their own, not as part of the curriculum.

A Life-Saving Relationship

As I moved back to Utah to finish my undergraduate degree, I moved in with my grandparents. It was wonderful to have a home cooked meal every day, but I largely subsisted on packaged cookies, rice crispy treats, chewy fruit candies, chocolate, and white rolls during the day while I was on campus. I also lived right next to a popular doughnuts shop, which didn't help matters. Though I tried to be healthier by eating fresh berries, making eggs each morning, juicing, and eating whole grain crackers, the effects of my binge eating offset any good I may have been doing by eating real foods.

Then one day, as fate would have it, while I was on a field trip with the BYU Political Affairs Society to the Utah State Capitol to meet with various Utah politicos, I sat next to a really good-looking young man on the bus. We instantly hit it off, and I knew that I was in love. We went on our first date a month later and, of course, went out for ice cream. As he would later confess, he would have asked me out earlier, but I told him I was a "vegetarian" in our first conversations. He figured he couldn't pursue a relationship with someone that didn't eat meat, so he didn't ask me out even though he wanted to. Though I was vegetarian, I ate plenty of processed and junk food to make up for any benefits I may have gained from not consuming meat. My new love interest, Jordan, seemed to notice and wanted to help me be healthier.

As we started dating, we would spend every spare moment together. On one occasion, in typical college fashion, we went late-night grocery shopping together. He bought apples, almond milk, cottage cheese, and granola. I had never seen a boy choose such healthy food before! I knew I had a winner, so when he proposed to me a few weeks later I instantly said yes. Our courtship was fast and furious. We started dating in April and were married by August. We were a match made in heaven, and there was no looking back. On one occasion, my mom pulled Jordan aside and, in his words, "asked if I was prepared to take on the load of health problems Cassidy had. She said that it was going to be a rocky road ahead and that Cassidy would be an expensive bride with rising medical costs." Even so, he wasn't deterred.

My love for Jordan was confirmed when he began taking care of me during bouts of severe illness. He took me to the ER a few times, and would often bring me food. He also would give me rides when my medications were kicking in, and I was unable to do so for myself. He had no problem ensuring I was home early, so I could get the sleep I needed. Just days before our wedding, from a growing concern for my health and with limited nutrition knowledge, he convinced me to begin eating meat again to ensure I had the proper nutrients and protein intake. He supported me completely in working through my health problems, but even then I'm sure he had little idea what he was getting himself into by marrying me. It wouldn't be until after we were married that either of us would fully grasp the gravity and severity of my health problems.

"You Could Die Young"

After getting married, we spent the first few months of our marriage living in Washington DC working as interns on Capitol Hill. My health problems persisted and even worsened to the point where I would miss work frequently. Living away from family also added a great deal of stress to my life. When we came home to resume our schooling, I had a laundry list of other issues to deal with aside from the stomach pains and extreme fatigue. I was missing a lot of work and school at this point, and it was unclear if I would ever be able to live a normal life. Still, I pressed forward and, with the help of my husband, looked all over for answers to my problems.

One Sunday evening after dinner with my in-laws, my mother-in-law recommended that I visit the functional medicine doctor they had been going to. He was naturally minded and preferred supplements and vitamins to medication when possible, though he still prescribed his fair share. He had been working with both my mother-in-law on her thyroid problems and my father-in-law for his Type 1 Diabetes and associated issues. I was excited to meet with him and give this new program a shot. I had tried the traditional medical route and wasn't feeling any better. In fact, things kept getting worse. I was open to any new suggestions and methods, so I immediately booked an appointment with their doctor.

When I first entered the office, they had me fill out extensive paperwork about all of my symptoms. As I handed the papers to the nurse who would ask questions and input everything into the system, she looked down and laughed. She looked back at me and said, "In all of my years as a nurse, I've never seen someone circle every single symptom on the page." She was mostly correct. I had circled every single symptom on the page except one. That was when I knew that I was in deep. The nurse drew what felt like ten gallons of blood, and I underwent other necessary tests to get more information on my worsening condition. I booked a follow-up appointment two weeks later and awaited more information.

As Jordan and I returned for the follow-up, I could tell the doctor and staff were very concerned. They handed me my paperwork and began to describe nearly a dozen conditions that had developed or were developing. In my journal I wrote, "I was diagnosed with about a million health conditions." Though exaggerated, I wasn't that far off. I was severely allergic to gluten. I had diabetic A1C levels. I had pre-lupus markers. I tested positive for arthritis. I had severe tendinitis. I had high cholesterol but extremely low blood pressure and many other diagnoses. The doctor then turned to me and very solemnly informed me that there were a lot of changes that I needed to make, but that I would likely die young. He told my husband to prepare for my early death and advised against having any children.

My life felt like it was shattering before my eyes and before it even really began! I couldn't die young! I had so many goals and plans for the future. The doctor's words sunk deep, and I don't remember much of anything else that day. Could this really be my life now? I had traded in my high heels and evening gowns for slippers and a hospital gown. The inflammation in my face was so bad, I was too embarrassed to have my picture taken. "How could this have happened to me?" I kept asking myself over and over. However, sitting in his office that day, I vowed to find an answer. From that moment, I embarked on a journey to find a cure for my laundry list of health problems. I wanted to discover for myself if food would play any kind of role. I just wasn't willing to accept that there weren't answers or solutions.

In what we thought was the answer, the doctor prescribed for me to immediately begin a keto diet and start on $700 worth of vitamins and supplements. I was willing to try anything and so, even as poor college students, we began the program that day. I remember buying my first pack of asparagus, and I felt like the healthiest person alive as I baked it with garlic that evening. I also bought Stevia, some berries, cheese, and a lot of grass-fed, organic meat. And by a lot, I mean a lot.

I started on the supplements and the new diet and started feeling better than I had in years. I had more energy, I wasn't as bloated, my stomach pain had lessened, and I even started losing some weight! Despite our additional $2000 a month in health expenses, I was sure I had found the answer to our problems. Our grocery budget went from $200/ month to over $1000. Additionally, my supplements were almost $700 a month as well, along with visits to the chiropractor and doctor. But I was encouraged because for the first time in years, I had seen my symptoms improve rather than worsen. I was convinced I had done the impossible and had saved myself. I was ready to proclaim the gospel of keto to the world.

Two Life-Changing Experiences

Going keto was hard but exciting for me. We transitioned to a steady animal product diet, with little-to-no processed or sugary foods in the home. For breakfast, I would make bacon and eggs. For lunch, we would often have chicken, raw cheese, or burgers. For dinner, I would make vegetables, meat, and a few berries. All of it was, of course, drenched in oils and fat, which I thought was the cure for my problems. I went all in on the paleo and keto train, and I was seeing results.

I managed to graduate from Brigham Young University with a B.A. in Political Science during this time. Shortly thereafter, I got my first job and was excited to be in the real world. With the stress of school off my shoulders, I had hoped that my health would improve. Though I was committed to eating keto at home, I would always sneak the forbidden foods at work. Despite my severe gluten allergies, I couldn't pass up a doughnut, and I would sneak a doughnut in a napkin and go in the hall to eat it so my coworkers wouldn't see. I would grab handfuls of various candies in the kitchen area and eat them throughout the day as well. I would always be in pain and suffer the consequences afterward, but I couldn't help myself.

During one project I ended up working 90-hour weeks and was completely overwhelmed. It was at this same time that I found out I was pregnant with our first child. I was elated, particularly because I had endured several miscarriages. I was also frightened about what the future would hold for this precious little human that I was growing. Though I was getting better, it was no shock to anyone who knew me that I was a long ways away from being "cured." I had more energy, but still had to retire by 8pm every night and sleep for 12 hours. My monthly bowel movements had improved, but I was still only having them once a week and continued to have blood in my stool. I had a long way to go before anyone would classify me as healthy.

It was during this time that I dug deeper and deeper into the world of nutrition. I did hours of research to find the best natural remedies for my conditions and to find foods that would help me heal. I had seen a glimmer of hope on the keto diet, and my whole body seemed to improve. I no longer felt like I was going to die, and I wanted to keep pushing and fighting until I was the healthiest person I knew. That was my goal–complete health.

After having a sausage and vegetable dinner one night, over a week and a half after my due date, I began to feel sick and then went into labor. My body wasn't quite ready to have this baby, but after getting food poisoning from our dinner, I had no choice. I spent the next 32 hours with fluids coming out both ends of my body. I was sad because the birthing experience ended up not being at all what I had envisioned, and it was ironically brought about by what I ate.

That's when God intervened and changed everything. One day, I had a seemingly random yet strong urge to go back to school to study nutrition. I researched every program and option and settled on getting a Master's and PhD through a distance learning program. Little did I know, that program would change the course of my life. Finding healing was just on the horizon, and I had no clue.

Doing the Unimaginable

When I began school, it was painstakingly obvious to me that animal products were very disruptive to health, something my own religion even taught.[9] I fought against that knowledge for some time before I considered that there might be something to it. Thousands of peer reviewed studies were telling me it was so, and it made me angry. I was eating a keto diet, and that's what I wanted to continue doing. For most of my life I had sought after worldly accolades and praise with great success, this made me a prideful person. I didn't easily admit that I was wrong, and I was both arrogant and haughty at times. However, I had been brought to the depths of humility as I struggled to even make it through each day. For the first time in my life, I was so unhappy and depressed. My successes meant nothing to me anymore. My crown meant nothing. My trophies and worldly pleasures meant nothing. By

God's grace I had been made so low, I had nowhere to look but up. As I began to consider ideas and information I had previously dismissed, I started to believe that there might be some hope. With all this information at my fingertips, it was time for me to act.

I knew I couldn't make a big dietary change on my own because of my struggles with food addiction, so I knew I needed to convince my husband to make the changes with me. Of course, he was just as skeptical (if not more) as I was. Thankfully, he wanted to support me, and we agreed to give this new way of eating a two-week trial. We often joke that we started our two-week trial and never ended it. Within days, I felt so incredible that I knew we couldn't go back. Bloating was gone. Heartburn was gone. Gas and other digestive problems were completely gone. My brain fog and depression began dissipating. My bowels started moving daily for the first time in my life! One of the greatest changes I noticed was with my addiction to food. I found that the more real foods I ate, the less I craved processed merchandise. At first, it was difficult and I would daydream about junk food. Over time, however, my taste buds changed. I was truly satiated after each meal for the first time in my life. I set hard and fast rules for myself, and I made the choice to never touch refined sugar again. This led me to find healthier alternatives such as dates or bananas to sweeten my foods.

Because of my studies on diet and nutrition, I was able to develop a plan for myself using the foods and herbs that I knew would best help to cleanse and heal my body. I spent many late nights and long hours fine-tuning my plan and I put my plan into action. My time studying paid off, and within weeks I was a new person. I put away my slippers, and traded them in for running shoes. Ironically, I had to throw away the only other pair of running shoes I had owned since I was thirteen–the shoes I had bought to wear on stage for my first national pageant. They got so little use that I was able to use them for over a decade with little wear and tear.

For the first time in my entire life I had enough energy to get up early in the morning and work out. I could do a full-work out with no issues–something that was previously impossible. I had so much energy I couldn't take a nap even if I tried! Everything was different; my skin glowed, my belly fat melted off, my eyes brightened, my hair got thicker and all this after having a baby! I looked and felt better than I ever did in the prime of my Miss Idaho days. But most importantly, for the very first time in my life, I felt happy. I wasn't winning pageants or any of the other stuff I used to do, but I was free. I was no longer a slave to my addictions and diseases. I was wearing my sweats all day long and looked like a homeless woman most days, but I didn't care one bit–I was finally happy!

Within months, I was 100% symptom free. In fact, when I went back to the doctor six months later for additional tests and blood work, the results came back completely clean. I had none of the indications of Crohn's disease nor any of the other problems I was previously diagnosed with. No inflammation, no bloating, no blood, no headaches, no kidney stones, no pain. My eyesight even improved, which my eye doctor said was extremely rare! The doctors were completely shocked as they gave me a clean bill of health. My health battle may have been won relatively easily, but it would take me years longer to defeat my food addiction and eating disorders–but that story deserves a book of its own.

Since that time, I have been among the healthiest people that I have ever encountered–somewhere I thought I would never be. Not only am I free from kidney stones, Crohn's disease, diabetes, and more, but I also don't fall prey to the common cold or the flu. On the rare occasions that I have contracted such an illness, it has only manifested minor symptoms like a stuffy nose and tiredness. My body is in proper working condition, and I have since birthed another beautiful baby in what one of my midwives suggested was "the healthiest pregnancy I've ever seen."

My life had been shiny, but completely fake–an illusion at best. I left that life for a dirt-filled, berry-stained mess, and I wouldn't trade it for the world! I haven't graced a stage in years, and heaven knows the last time I put on a pair of high heels. But the joy I feel from working in the garden or sprouting buckwheat with my kids is unparalleled. I haven't needed any big wins to feel happy, because I found that when I ate real foods and connected to my food sources, I became more real. Nearly every aspect of my life has been changed, and I owe it all to food.

What I did to heal myself is not revolutionary or some big, ancient secret. All I did was trade in my processed, manufactured lifestyle for a simple and natural one. It was finding the right foods in the right order that made all the difference. In the rest of the book I'll tell you exactly what I did.

Chapter Three

The IBD Reversal Diet

According to the Crohn's and Colitis Foundation 2019 Factbook, remission of any kind using the typically prescribed route of drugs and surgery is around 30 percent for both Crohn's disease and ulcerative colitis.[10] They suggest the relapse rate for Crohn's is 76 percent.[11] This means that over three-fourths of all those who get the disease have no hope for permanent or lasting remission! Lifestyle changes, such as the ones discussed in this book, are not even mentioned in this factbook. This unfortunate state of affairs is echoed by an IBD in America Survey from 2017, which revealed that only 33 percent of respondents were at any point in remission, and three-fourths of that 33 percent were in remission for less than 3 years.[12] Of those in remission, medication was still required by 77 percent!

What if I told you there were peer reviewed medical journals that housed dozens of studies indicating it is possible to achieve 100 percent remission rate? Would you believe me if I said that there is data to suggest you can be entirely medication free and still be in remission? What if I said you could feel better than you ever have your entire life by making a few lifestyle changes?

When I was diagnosed with Crohn's disease, my whole world was turned upside down. No one seemed to know what to do or how to find relief, and I was essentially told this diagnosis would be my new life. When I went back to school for a PhD and began studying nutrition more in depth, I started implementing what I learned. Over time, I found that there were certain foods that helped to heal and build the gut and ones that did not. Through a lot of research, trial, and error, I came up with what I termed the "IBD Reversal Diet." This is what I used to heal my gut, and I have seen this type of diet heal many others who suffer from IBD, IBS, and many other lifestyle diseases. Because each person's situation is different, I have broken up the diet into four simple principles. Adherence to each principle is crucial for success and must be done in the right order to see the long-term desired results.

Principle #1: Cleanse the Body

The first principle to heal from any disease is to cleanse the body of toxins. Cleansing the body ought to be done before any other steps are taken. Each day of our lives we are exposed to toxins. According to the Environmental Protection Agency (EPA), there are over 595 common toxins that cause significant health damage in humans.[13] As Dr. Leigh Erin Connealy, author of The Cancer Revolution, said, "[Toxins] may come from the chemicals in the air, electromagnetic field radiation from your cell phones, processed food that you eat and so on".[14] Indeed, we eat these toxins, we drink them, and we breathe them in.

In 2010, the Centers for Disease Control and Prevention (CDC) conducted the Fourth National Report on Human Exposure to Environmental Chemicals. In this report they found over 212 chemicals in participants' bodies via their urine or blood.[15] A staggering 75 of these had never before been found in the human body. Some chemicals include formaldehyde, jet fuel, and many more. This bioaccumulation of toxins is linked with brain and nervous system malfunction, and autoimmune disease.[16] It would be nearly impossible to suggest that our genetic expressions and subsequent health are not dramatically impacted by the constant exposure to these toxins.

With such high levels of exposure to toxins, it is absolutely necessary to purge our bodies of the accumulations that have built up over time and have inhibited our bodies from performing their natural functions. The good news is you don't need a fancy spa, expensive and rare supplements, or an intricate plan to cleanse! Cleansing can take place by simply using foods. When toxins build up in the body, disease can take root. When our immune systems are working on overdrive trying to fight off the McDonald's we had for lunch, there is no bandwidth left to work on healing our autoimmune conditions. Therefore, the first and perhaps easiest toxins to eliminate are the ones found in food. Get rid of the toxic foods and begin taking in healing foods. There will be immediate and noticeable changes.

It may surprise you to learn that our digestive system is the second largest part of the neurological system. Many are certainly surprised to learn that 80 percent of the entire immune system is found there! Microbes in the digestive tract that make up the gut flora are responsible for an incredible amount of processes, which, if deficient, are linked to nearly all autoimmune diseases.[17] This should lead us to reason that if the digestive system is so important, it surely needs more cleansing from built up toxins than anywhere else in the body.

Interestingly enough, in 1999, an estimated 66 million Americans suffered from chronic constipation.[18] Surely, that number is much higher today. In fact, anyone who is not having 3-4 bowel movements a day does not have a proper functioning digestive system. Having these consistent bowel movements is crucial to digestive health. When many people hear of constipation, they think of few and very hard bowel movements. While this is true, constipation can be found anywhere in the digestive tract and may not always be associated with difficult bowel movements. Many are surprised to learn that you can be constipated and still have severe diarrhea. Further still, the cause of diarrhea is usually constipation. In my time helping people with chronic disease, I have found in nearly every case that when you can get rid of constipation, the disease can also disappear. The best way to eliminate constipation is through cleansing and proper nutrition.

There are many ways to cleanse, and some are more safe and effective than others. But it is important to remember that during this phase, we are not building the gut flora yet. There should be no probiotics or gut building foods. This phase is simply for healing the gut lining, so simple and easily digested foods should be the only ones consumed during this phase. This means that lightly cooked or steamed foods should be the focus. While later in the cleanse we will focus on raw foods, now is a time to *avoid* raw.

For those that I have worked with and myself, starches have proven the most effective in the initial cleansing phase. This comes as no surprise, because studies show that many starches are extremely beneficial for colon health.[19] The particular starches that I have seen effective are brown rice and potatoes of all varieties. These are best utilized when cooked at low temperatures, and when the brown rice is soaked and sprouted. I've seen incredible results from people using primarily these foods. However, some may also choose to utilize small amounts of other gluten-free grains such as quinoa, buckwheat, millet, and amaranth. In some cases, incredible things happen within hours of adjusting a diet to focus on these foods. As Dr. John McDougall points out,

> "Bowel contents must be changed continually in order to get long lasting significant improvement. The simple increase of the fiber content in the foods eaten has been shown to reduce the frequency of attacks and to improve symptoms in many patients. A starch-based diet, which is inherently high in fiber, is highly effective at alleviating the distress from this condition."[20]

Along with the starches, steamed and lightly cooked vegetables such as squash, green peas, carrots, green beans, mushrooms, and other similar vegetables are very helpful. Because cooked vegetables are easier on digestion, these are also very helpful during an initial cleansing period. These vegetables provide a number of important nutrients to the digestive tract, which is a crucial step since those suffering from IBD are usually malnourished as well.[21] For example, squash is high in omega 3 fatty-acids and antioxidants including zeaxanthin, lutein, and beta-carotene. Eating a greater amount of these will not only be easier on digestion but will provide vital nutrients to aid the body in healing. Small amounts of tofu and cooked fruit can be eaten if tolerated as well. As we will discuss later, animal products, sugar, processed foods and gluten should be avoided from here on out as well.

This first phase of healing can take anywhere from two weeks to six months depending on the person. But ultimately, you know you are ready to add additional foods back in when you have 3-4 well-formed bowel movements, with no blood or pain each day.

There is one point regarding vegetables I want to caution on, however. When someone is in a flare-up or experiencing other severe problems, even the best of foods like dark leafy greens can cause pain. Because of this, many people benefit from forgoing these foods for a short period of time to focus on starches and allow the digestive system a short break from the hard work it has been doing! When cleansing on these foods, it is most effective when no other foods are taken but the ones mentioned above. This allows the digestive system ample nutrients and resources to heal itself during this cleansing phase. This, however, does not need to be a long term solution. Foods such as dark leafy greens ought to constitute a good portion of our diet.

Another important part of cleansing is drinking plenty of pure water. Water is incredibly important to nearly every process and function in your body. The kidneys, liver, and other organs require water to cleanse blood, produce urine, and help the body to get rid of waste. Unfortunately, today's water is contaminated with nearly 300 forms of neurotoxins, carcinogens, endocrine disruptors, heavy metals, and more.[22] Even though many of these are legal in small doses, it doesn't mean they are safe. According to the Environmental Working Group, the standards for tap water haven't been updated in over 20 years, and many chemicals that are currently allowed in our water have been proven to be unsafe.[23] As you can imagine, these chemicals are wreaking havoc on our health.

While it is clear that it is incredibly important to filter your water, there is some debate about which water filtration is best. Ultimately the choice is yours, but the cleanest and best water source I am aware of is distilled water. Distilled water helps to remove the harmful toxins and minerals while moving the good, health-promoting minerals to the proper places in the body. If this isn't an option for you, just do the best you can in ensuring that you can get filtered water. Once you have the right kind of water, increase your water intake each day so that you are drinking enough to flush out the toxic accumulations through the bowels.

This first step of cleansing is very important and should not be overlooked. When we have years worth of accumulated toxins and dead matter, we will not make much progress in getting well until the body is cleaned out. Some of my clients have reported that their symptoms worsen initially in this cleansing phase. They report abdominal pain, nausea, extreme fatigue, diarrhea, etc. These symptoms are expected for a cleanse, as it's pulling out toxins which can be an intense process. But do not worry or quit if you experience these symptoms, things will get better. Cleansing can be a roller coaster and sometimes we have to go lower before we can go higher. For some, this may take longer than it will for others, but most of those I have worked with have reported feeling better than ever after completing a cleanse. And the good news is that it's only the first step.

Step 2: Find the Right Herbs

Alongside cleansing the body, herbs are extremely helpful in achieving long-term relief and healing. Many mainstream doctors will tell you that herbs are unsafe. This is true; there *are* herbs that are unsafe. However, there are many herbs that have been used for thousands of years for healing the gut. We are just now beginning to scientifically understand their effectiveness. In fact, you might be surprised to learn that in head-to-head trials researchers have routinely found that herbs outperform modern medicine. One study found that ashwagandha was more effective than hydrocortisone at reducing inflammation.[24] Chamomile has been shown to treat ulcers and lower acidity in the stomach more than antacids.[25] Passionflower is found to be as equally effective as oxazepam (Serax) for treating anxiety.[26] The list goes on, but the idea remains the same. When it comes to dealing with a health problem, there is often an herb that can perform the same function as its doctor-prescribed counterpart.

So what herbs are ideal for IBD? Ultimately, it's best to consult about your specific situation with one who is knowledgeable about the historic and safe use of herbs in the body, because various herbs can have different effects based on individual conditions and medications. However, numerous studies have shown incredible results for all kinds of herbs in healing both IBD and IBS.

Boswellia is typically known for its sweet smelling resins that are often used in oils. However, many are unaware that it is an extremely effective aid for IBD. One study found that 70 percent of patients who used

Boswellia achieved remission, significantly outperforming medication.[27] Another study showed similar results, showing significantly greater results from Boswellia than sulfasalazine.[28] It has also been shown to aid in preventing colitis.[29]

Turmeric is one herb that is extremely beneficial for any form of digestive disorder. One study found that colitis patients had a 50 percent higher remission rate when using turmeric than those who did not use it.[30] Turmeric is also associated with a 60 percent reduction in pain and a 73 percent reduction in joint stiffness.[31] This kind of incredible relief is likely because turmeric contains "curcumin," a property that fights oxidative damage and boosts the body's own antioxidant enzymes.[32] Curcumin has been found to be anti-inflammatory, anti-cancer, anti-amyloid, antioxidant, anti-microbial and anti-arthritic.[33] No wonder it has been shown to effectively aid in dealing with most autoimmune diseases, including IBD.[34] Some studies even suggest it performs these functions better than leading medications![35]

In Europe, slippery elm is a popular and extremely effective treatment for IBD.[36] Some say that slippery elm is nature's mesalamine, without any of the side effects. It has been shown to be a wonderful treatment for IBD, in part because of its antioxidant effects on the cells.[37] Many claim that it is one of the best herbs out there for soothing the digestive tract. It is one of my personal favorites for an upset stomach of any kind. It has also been shown to greatly improve symptoms of IBS.[38]

Licorice root is also an incredible anti-inflammatory herb that has been shown to be quite an effective remedy for colitis.[39] It has proven effective in fighting against nausea, indigestion, and stomach pain.[40] Perhaps one of the greatest benefits is its anti-ulcer properties that make it an incredible aid for many forms of IBD and IBS.[41] Licorice root is recommended by many natural minded physicians to help soothe the digestive tract.

While there are many additional herbs that I have seen bring tremendous success, you get the picture. Herbs can and do heal–even herbs we never would have imagined. For instance, people are often shocked to learn that cayenne is extremely beneficial for IBD and IBS, helping to significantly reduce symptoms.[42] For me, cayenne was a game changer! I noticed that within days of taking it, the blood in my stool was completely gone and my ulcer pain went away. When it comes down to it, herbs can be an essential part of healing IBD or any autoimmune disease! It may sound too good to be true to find a plant that is just as effective in trials for a fraction of the cost of medication, but I assure you this

is real life. As one of my clients once said, "What did I
ever do before herbs?"

Step 3: Build the Gut

After cleansing the body and starting to use helpful
herbs, it's time to build the gut flora and focus on the
right kinds of foods. When you think of building the
gut flora, you likely think of using probiotics because
this is the usual first step many doctors take, both
alternative and conventional. However, recent studies
suggest that probiotics aren't as effective or helpful as
previously thought.[43] This makes sense given that
probiotics are made in a laboratory and are not
naturally occurring. Moreover, while these bottled
probiotics boast something like 100 million strains of
probiotic, what they don't tell you is that 1 strain is
usually replicated 100 million times. So while you are
anticipating getting a wide variety of bacterial strains,
you only come out with five or six.

That is to say nothing of the studies indicating that
probiotics often increase histamines in the body, leading
to blood vessel damage and associated symptoms.[44]
Perhaps the most concerning study was a comparative
study looking at the impacts of antibiotics, probiotics,
and a fecal transplant. This study revealed that
probiotics killed the gut flora more than antibiotics and
delayed recovery time significantly.[45] These shocking

results put into perspective just how harmful probiotics can be, especially if antibiotics (which are notorious for harming gut flora) are less damaging than probiotics.

But all hope is not lost! Though a bottled probiotic is not beneficial, there are many probiotic-rich foods that are. According to Dr. Natasha Campbell-McBride, a single serving (one teaspoon) of fermented vegetables has more beneficial bacteria than an entire bottle of a high potency probiotic product![46] Foods like miso, kimchi, sauerkraut, pickles, kefir, rejuvelac, apple cider vinegar and kombucha are welcome additions to a recovering gut flora.

Experiment with these foods and see which ones work for you. It is important that these foods are not cooked and are as natural as possible. That is why it can often be beneficial to buy them both raw and organic, or make them yourself. You will find that over time you will begin to really enjoy these foods. For instance, my toddler would beg for sauerkraut every day and eat it plain from a bowl! However you decide to do it, these foods ought to be a central part of your recovery.

In my opinion, the best part about this phase is that you can start eating living foods again! This is a relief, especially because a meta analysis found significantly lower rates of IBD in people who ate large quantities of fruits and vegetables.[47] Additionally, a number of studies show that many foods play an incredibly important role in IBD healing. For instance, broccoli builds the intestinal lining.[48] Also, dark leafy greens are the best source of folate, or B9, an essential nutrient for healthy cell division.[49]

The key to this step, as I have already touched on, is avoiding processed laboratory foods and eating unadulterated, real foods. Munch on a satiating mango from the tree. Luxuriate in a ripe raspberry right from the cane. Coat your taste buds in a carrot picked fresh from the ground. No work or processing necessary, just real foods providing the highest nutrient value on the planet! They are better for you than any "super food supplement" made in a lab. Nothing can ever outperform nature's wonders. Eat these foods as close to their natural state as possible and forgo cooking when you are able.

Raw foods are incredibly healthy for every part of your body and ought to make up a majority of the calories consumed from this point on. Raw foods have many benefits, but most important are their enzymes. Since our bodies' metabolic and digestive enzymes are finite, it is crucial to supplement with food enzymes so that the chemical processes in our body can function properly. Unfortunately, food enzymes, which are found in all fruits, vegetables, grains, nuts and seeds, are killed in any heat over 118°F.[50] These foods must be uncooked to reap the benefits of their enzymes. Since phytonutrients don't stand up well to heat, many antioxidant foods lose their valuable properties by cooking them.[51] And wouldn't you know it, these raw foods have also been shown to be an incredible aid for IBD.[52] Therefore, it is ideal to incorporate more raw foods in any long term diet.

Fruits are essential to healing any autoimmune condition, but particularly IBD. One study found that citrus was extremely protective against colitis.[53] Yet another study found that eating black raspberries protected against ulcers.[54] Just in 2020, a groundbreaking study found that blueberries were an effective treatment for IBD.[55] Bananas improve digestion and increase good gut flora.[56] The list could go on and on. Fruits are an incredible source of healing for us and ought to be eaten freely in the recovery phase and for the rest of one's life.

As excited as we can be to get back to raw foods after the cleansing period, it should be done carefully and with caution. That means that you should only add foods back in at the rate of one new food per day. This allows the body time to adjust and slowly introduce new minerals, vitamins, bacteria and other nutrients into the body in a way that will not overwhelm it after it has undergone a cleansing period. For example, on Monday I would add in avocados, Tuesday I could add in spinach, Wednesday I could add in strawberries, etc.

Throughout the next few weeks your diet will slowly transition to the right kinds of foods to build the gut flora again and you will be well on your way to permanently healing the intestinal lining.

Throughout time you will come to love juicing, smoothies, salads, and even just fruit bowls! These foods will help to build the microbes that have been destroyed through medication, candida, or cleansing. This process can be jump-started with a short weekend juicing cleanse, which is something I found extremely effective for myself and a number of clients.

Step 4: Avoid Toxins

Once you cleanse and begin building the gut flora back up, it's incredibly important to reduce inflammation and allow the intestines to function at their best. Surprising to some is that animal products are at the very top of the list of toxic foods. A plant based diet has been found, time and time again, to be the most superior treatment to, not only IBD, but other autoimmune conditions as well. It is therefore very important for those wishing to heal from IBD or IBS to avoid animal products long term.

This isn't some alternative or quack perspective; there is overwhelming data to support this claim. The Physicians Committee for Responsible Medicine simply said that a plant based diet is "unreservedly recommended for IBD."[57] The studies that support this are astounding! One study found that relapse rates of those eating a plant based diet were 0 percent at one year and 8 percent at two years. Conversely, the relapse rates of those on an omnivorous diet were 33 percent after one year and 75 percent after two years.[58] Numerous other studies have produced the same results: a 100 percent remission rate on a plant based diet.[59] A 100 percent remission rate is mind blowing when you consider that the Crohn's and Colitis Foundation asserts that "between 66 and 75 percent of Crohn's disease patients will require surgery at some point."[60] Moreover, patients who use both surgery and combination therapy (infliximab and azathioprine) reach a remission rate of about 50 percent.[61] If we believe these incredible dietary studies, a whole new world of hope opens up!

I know this is hard to hear for many people, but instances of IBD are consistently linked with high meat consumption.[62] Eating meat not only increases your risk of getting Crohn's, but it also increases the severity of symptoms.[63] This association between meat and Crohn's is not minimal. For many, including myself, getting rid of meat got rid of my symptoms almost immediately. It should come as no surprise then, that one of the strongest dietary factors for Crohn's and colitis is meat consumption.[64] Complete remission is the goal for each patient, and though a plant based diet boasts 100 percent remission rate, studies have found that relapse rates are highest among those who eat meat.[65] For me, this knowledge was enough to pull me away from my beloved bacon, and perhaps it will motivate you to do the same as well.

Speaking anecdotally, I have seen dramatic improvements within 24 hours of stopping eating any meat products. When the intestines are allowed time to reduce inflammation and begin healing, marvelous benefits come. I often compare having IBD or IBS to falling and scraping your knee. When you fall and skin your knee, there is an immediate inflammatory response from your body. That response is intended to protect the newly formed wound which is open and prime for infection. The body responds by sending all of its available resources to help heal the wound. This is just like our intestines. When we get any bowel disorder of any kind, our intestines are essentially an open wound. That open wound is eager to heal, and sends all available resources to the area. Continuing with this analogy, if you go home after scraping your knee and put a bandaid on it, neglecting to wash, disinfect, and clear it out, there is sure to be more trouble. Moreover, if you take no precautions and continue to fall on that same skinned knee day after day, that scrape will never have time to heal over and you will be left with perpetual knee problems for the rest of your life. Similarly, after getting IBD, if you continue to eat the same inflammatory foods every single day, never allowing the intestines time to heal over or build a protective lining, you will be left with perpetual intestinal problems. Your intestines and colon will never have time to heal over. The inflammatory foods continue to exacerbate the problem, not allowing these digestive organs time to heal.

With this in mind, some may wonder if a plant based diet is beneficial for other diseases, and the answer is YES! Studies indicate 50 percent less hyperthyroidism among those who eat a plant based diet compared to those who eat omnivorous diets. An 18-year study found a strong correlation between overconsumption of protein and increased risk of diabetes. The results showed a 7,300 percent increased risk of developing diabetes on an animal protein diet.[66] A 1970s study involving 20 countries found that multiple sclerosis (MS) was directly associated with meat, eggs, milk, butter, and sugar intake.[67] This led world-famous Dr. Swank to declare a plant based diet as "the most effective treatment of multiple sclerosis ever reported in the peer review literature."[68] These are just a few examples, but the list goes on and on. The studies are clear–a plant based diet is ideal for every single condition, including every form of IBS (IBD's less severe counterpart).

Though removing meat is a good start, it is important to remove all animal products to get true healing. Dairy is often more of an issue than meat for certain people. Some research suggests that colitis may be caused by an allergic reaction to dairy.[69] Other studies have found that Ulcerative Colitis patients experienced dramatically less symptoms by removing dairy and nearly all of them had severe symptoms return when dairy was added back in.[70] Similarly, Crohn's symptoms have also been directly linked to dairy as well.[71]

In addition to dairy, things like eggs shouldn't be consumed by individuals with IBD, either. Over 60 percent of the total calories in an egg are from fat.[72] Fat is one of the primary contributors to developing IBD. Eggs have specifically been linked with increased risk of IBD.[73] One landmark study took Crohn's patients that had severe diarrhea (20+ bowel movements per day) and switched their diet to low fat. Within two to three days most patients had relief.[74] Additionally, eggs are associated with a plethora of other ills including heart disease,[75] diabetes,[76] and cancer.[77] Clearly, animal products ought to be avoided regardless of which health condition you may have.

Now you may be wondering, what about bone broth? Dr. Axe and Dr. Mercola, among other "gut specialists," strongly recommend taking bone broth to improve gut health and heal the intestinal lining. However, there is no evidence showing bone broth to be effective. The first study on bone broth concluded that it was a poor source of most nutrients.[78] Bone broth has also been found to be extremely high in lead.[79] In an article titled 'Science can't explain why everyone is drinking bone broth,' Dr. William H. Percy (professor, biomedical scientist, professor and researcher) says, "The idea that because bone broth or stock contains collagen it somehow translates to collagen in the human body is nonsensical. Collagen is actually a pretty poor source of amino acids."[80] Perhaps the most concerning aspect of bone broth is it's link to "leaky brain." In an attempt to solve leaky gut, we take bone broth which is full of glutamic acid.[81] Glutamic acid is an excitotoxin that, in excess, can bypass the blood brain barrier and cause a number of grave complications.[82] Ultimately, bone broth isn't as healing as many think.

On this topic of animal products, we could argue that there is "data on both sides" as I so often hear, but the proof is in the pudding–plant based pudding, of course. I have yet to meet a single person in my years of working with IBD that has permanently achieved remission or reversed their problems while using animal products. On the contrary, I have met many who were promised healing but were met with pain and heartache using animal products. I have, however, aided numerous individuals as they found hope and healing for the first time since their diagnosis by omitting all animal products. For some, this is the biggest and most crucial step in healing their digestive woes.

After animal foods, the next items that ought to be entirely eliminated are refined sugar products. Research has linked sugar and artificial sweeteners to IBD.[83] Refined sugar in all forms impairs immune function and significantly harms white blood cells.[84] Each bite of sugar we take suppresses our immune response, exacerbating the impacts of IBD drastically. Unsurprisingly, sugar is linked to worsening autoimmune disease due to its inflammatory nature.[85] With these things in mind, it is pretty clear that sugar must be eliminated. Now before you mourn over never being able to have a dessert again, know there are plenty of healthy alternatives like dates, figs, maple syrup and honey. In many cases I sweeten foods with apples and bananas! These natural sweeteners can be used in moderation without producing the same effects as processed sweeteners, and I have yet to meet anyone who doesn't like my healthy desserts.

The next thing that many are surprised to learn about is gluten products. Crohn's patients are more genetically predisposed to gluten intolerance and Celiac, making it an important food to avoid.[86] Not only do gluten products make you more likely to get the disease, but it worsens symptoms. Over 65 percent of patients who went gluten-free reported fewer symptoms and flares.[87] This is confirmed by another study that showed that patients who removed gluten from their diet had improved symptoms.[88] Gluten products, while often turned to as a comfort food, can be the cause of so much woe in IBD! However, substituting with foods like oats or buckwheat can be very easy. In one study, oat bran proved effective in maintaining remission and also showed a significant increase in butyrate, a short-chain fatty acid that is known to heal the intestinal wall.[89] Some of my clients have found that using ancient grains such as spelt, einkorn, kamut, and others have not yielded the same inflammatory responses. Though it would depend on the individual, you may consider experimenting with one of the many ancient grains options available as an alternative.

Again, I completely understand how difficult this might be for some people. Animal products, sugar and gluten are highly addictive and are often what we use to numb difficult emotions we don't want to deal with.

I was there at one point. I was once addicted to ice cream, cheese and eggs in all their forms. But I can confidently say that the amount of relief and healing that will come by giving up these harmful products will far outweigh any personal appetites for them.

In Summary

Though it may seem complex, the major components to the IBD Reversal Diet can be summarized in these four simple principles. Obviously each case is different and needs adjusting and personalization to find the right balance, which is why I always recommend working with a professional to do it the right way and fine tune each piece of the puzzle. If that isn't an option for you, start here and master these main points.

Principle 1: Cleanse the Body
- There are many toxins in our environment and bodies
- It is important to cleanse frequently and correctly
- Eat only easily digested foods like starches for a short period of time
- Drink clean water

Principle 2: Find the Right Herbs

- Herbs often outperform drugs in head-to-head trials
- Consult a skilled professional to find the best option for you and your situation
- There are many great herbs for IBD. A few of them include:
  - Turmeric
  - Boswellia
  - Slippery elm
  - Licorice root
  - Cayenne

Principle 3: Build the Gut

- Bottled probiotics are NOT your friends. Opt for probiotic-rich foods
- Eat as many uncooked, unprocessed and real foods as possible

Principle 4: Permanently Avoid Toxins

- Stop meat, dairy, and eggs ASAP
  - Plant based diets are associated with 100 percent remission rates
- Bone broth isn't as good as it's marketed to be
- Refined sugar contributes to autoimmune disease
- Gluten intolerance is common among IBD and IBS

Though these are the primary steps one should take, they are certainly not the only things that ought to be done to heal IBD or other autoimmune problems. I would be remiss if I didn't address a few of the other lifestyle factors that contribute as well. For example, one study done in the Netherlands found that 82 percent of IBD patients were vitamin D deficient.[90] While it is clear that diet plays a role in vitamin D absorption, using the above steps is sufficient along with daily sun exposure to manage this deficiency. Studies also link stress to IBD flares.[91] Therefore, stress management techniques prove very beneficial to many dealing with both IBD and IBS. This can include things like daily exercise, journaling, prayer, affirmations, relationship management, and more. As you find your weak points and work to improve, you will notice big changes.

I once had a client who, despite eating perfectly and following the program, continued to have flare-ups. During one appointment she broke into tears, telling me that she was in an abusive relationship and each time they got in a fight, she had a flare-up. Her problems persisted until she ended the relationship and got the help she needed. After seeking help, her symptoms disappeared. It's important to remember that IBD is a lifestyle disease, and sometimes it takes more than just food to get to the bottom of the problem.

A Few Reminders

That's it! With these principles you can take back your life and get on the road to health and healing. I know, because I have been there myself. It's amazing what four lifestyle changes can do to your body. It opens doors that you never thought were possible. It can truly be the difference of a lifetime. There is nothing more rewarding than gaining control of your life and doing things you never thought possible, like plan a night out without grabbing the seat nearest to the bathroom.

Though it may seem easy, this kind of approach to IBD and health takes work. Some days you'll feel like giving up. I had one client who continually told me that she hated me and that I was her best friend at the same time. It's a difficult road, and cleansing is not an easy process. It is sometimes accompanied by discomfort and pain, both physical and emotional. As your body heals, it can be a real whirlwind. When I got healthy, I noticed an influx of very difficult emotions flood over me as years of suppressed feelings came to the surface. This has been reported by nearly every one of my clients. So, along with traditional detox symptoms, also be on the lookout for emotional detoxing as well and realize it's both normal and healthy to be experiencing these things. Thankfully, I had someone to support me throughout all of the difficulties that came up. I would absolutely recommend having someone you can count on when things get tough as you start to heal your body.

Another thing I see is that many people will get complacent. They work hard by eating the right foods, taking the right herbs, and giving themselves the care they need. After they feel better, they don't experience the same pain and restrictions they did before, so it's easy to fall off the bandwagon. Over time they begin sneaking tiny bits of processed foods or oil; they have small amounts of dairy or sugar. Before they know it, they are bloated and their inflammation increases again.

Eating this way is a lifetime endeavor. It's a commitment to eat real food and shun the denatured and processed foods. When we do this, we see the results. When we falter, we feel the impacts. I, myself, have had times of weakness when I gave in to processed "vegan foods." Though I worked hard to stay clear of animal products, I started feeling fatigued and bloated again due to the foods I had let sneak into my diet. The change happens so slowly and imperceptibly it's hard to notice sometimes. That is why I recommend tracking your food intake for the first little while using a food journal, and doing so again for a few days every three to four months. This helps you to stay on track and watch for any unhealthy foods or habits that may have snuck into your new lifestyle.

I know this is not easy. When it's all said and done, though you may sacrifice some of your favorite foods now, it brings more freedom in the long run. It certainly is a lot of work and effort to make these changes! Some days are more difficult than others and if you're anything like me you'll shed a few tears along the way. Saying no to your favorite shrimp tacos might seem unbearable, but it's a sacrifice worth making. Imagine no more bleeding, no more pain and bloating, no more trips to the bathroom, energy to do all of your favorite activities again. These things are possible when we do what it takes to heal. For me, it was absolutely worth it, and in a later chapter, you'll hear from others who changed their lives with this diet!

Chapter Four

Overcoming Food Addiction

When I set out to write this book, I didn't plan on writing a section on food addiction. Throughout the writing process, however, I kept feeling like something was missing. It soon dawned on me that food addiction played just as big a role in my story as Crohn's disease did. Additionally, a vast majority of my clients suffer from food addiction, which, as I can attest, makes IBD even more difficult. Food addiction is so prevalent that one study found 92 percent of people have some form of food addiction. So, I would be remiss to not address it in this book.

Kicking Addictive Foods

The first aspect of food addiction worth consideration is the addictive nature of food itself. Much of the merchandise passed as food on supermarket shelves today are full of preservatives, fillers, and chemicals! These products were often made with the intent to be addicting. Their whole purpose is to make us come back for more. The manufacturers of these products have done a pretty good job of enticing us back for more–fast food chains made over 230 billion dollars in 2020, despite the Coronavirus pandemic.[92] But the addictive nature of these foods is not just some ethereal thing. We can actually measure it.

Years ago, Yale created a model to measure food addiction called the "Yale Food Addiction Scale (YFAS)."[93] This model has been used to determine the presence and extent of someone's food addiction. Many studies have been done based on this model. One study set out to determine the most and least addictive foods according to the YFAS model.[94] The findings are fascinating and were reported on a scale of 1-7, 1 being least addictive and 7 being most addictive. The most addictive foods were:

- pizza (4.01)
- chocolate (3.73)
- chips (3.73)
- cookies (3.71)
- ice cream (3.68)
- french fries (3.60)
- cheeseburgers (3.51)
- soda (not diet) (3.29)
- cake (3.26)
- cheese (3.22)

- bacon (3.03)
- fried chicken (2.97)
- rolls (plain) (2.73)
- popcorn (buttered) (2.64)
- breakfast cereal (2.59)
- gummy candy (2.57)
- steak (2.54)
- muffins (2.50)

You may notice that none of these foods are included in my IBD Reversal Diet. That's not by accident. The above mentioned foods contain no nutritional value, especially when dealing with chronic gastrointestinal troubles! Moreover, they are unfit for us mentally. As we avoid the very foods that keep drawing us in for more, we can begin our healing process. But the study didn't stop there. It also discovered the least addictive foods. Some of which are:

- cucumbers (1.53)
- carrots (1.60)
- beans (no sauce) (1.63)
- apples (1.66)
- brown rice (1.74)
- broccoli (1.74)
- bananas (1.77)
- corn (no butter or salt) (1.87)

- strawberries (1.88)
- granola bar (1.93)
- water (1.94)
- crackers (plain) (2.07)

Getting rid of the addictive foods is the first step in overcoming food addiction. The dopamine created from eating the addictive foods lights up the pleasure centers of the brain.[95] The reward in the brain is much higher for eating processed foods than from eating fruits and vegetables, which keeps us coming back for more.[96] The more dopamine that is released when we eat, the more we want that food. The pleasure is only temporary so it's not long enough to sustain us. We have to keep eating more and more just to feel as good as we did for 20 seconds after the first bite. Before you know it an entire box of Oreos is gone and you still aren't satisfied. When you think about it, our brains are being hijacked and manipulated for the profit margins of the corporations who manufacture those addictive products.

However, the naturally occurring fruits and vegetables do not light up the same pleasure centers of the brain. Because of this, they don't feel as rewarding at first. We may not even like them because we are so used to the intense dopamine release that makes us feel good. We may even go through withdrawals, but over time, your brain quits expecting the same release and is content with the less addictive foods. This inherently lessens the addiction. Changing diet is the best way to break the cycle. You can control what you put in your mouth, even if you can't control everything else in your life.

For the food addict, the best answer is to abandon those foods altogether. I know this may be easier said than done, but replacing the standard American diet with a diet high in fruits, vegetables, and whole grains is a huge step in the right direction. Allowing yourself to eat substantial amounts of fruits and vegetables is healthy both physically and mentally. Rather than restrict or calorie count, eating real foods allows you the freedom to continue to eat plenty of food to suffice your needs. It simultaneously retrains your brain and stomach to turn to food only for fuel for your bodies and not for emotional coping. You can fill your stomach with satiating foods, and soon your cravings will begin to subside as your health and vitality increase.

This sentiment may be true, but I have often heard that it is easier to change one's religion than it is to change one's diet. Changing one's diet is an incredibly difficult process if you look at the big picture. Stop eating all chips, candy, soda, sugar, dairy, yogurt, milk, cheese, eggs, meat, pizza, chocolate, and anything else that's pleasurable and eat boring bland vegetables the rest of your life? Many people look at it this way and it's no wonder they are overwhelmed by the process!

However, I believe that eating healthy is one of the easiest changes you can make in your life because you can take it one bite at a time. Your diet consists of hundreds of small changes each day, not one large choice. That means that if you mess up, you have the next bite to rectify your mistake. Each bite that you take into your mouth is a new choice, and it's one that is manageable. You can begin by making each bite count. Instead of pumping yourself full of pizza, opt for a nice large apple and savor each bite. Eat slowly and methodically, thoroughly masticate, and let food truly become your friend, not your enemy.

One exercise that I have my clients do is mindful eating. As they sit down to eat, I have them look at their plate and take 30 seconds to admire it. Look at the colors, textures, and patterns. Consider where that food might have come from, where it was grown, the soil it was made in. Think of the care that brought it to you and what it took to get it from the store to your plate. With thankfulness, take each bite slowly and enjoy every burst of flavor. This is truly how we make each bite count. In our busy world of fast food and entertainment, we just shove whatever is in front of us into our mouths with no thought. This is where food addiction begins, separating ourselves from our food choices. If we dial in and connect with our food, we will begin to see magnificent changes.

Address Underlying Emotional Needs

I wish I could say that just eating better would take care of all food addiction, but it won't. Throughout my entire life I turned to food to numb the emotional pain and stress in my life. I was completely unfilled and miserable, and food was my drug of choice. Eventually those emotions grew so big that it took over my body and manifested itself in disease. The whole time I had underlying emotional needs that had not been met. It has been said that we carry the world on our plate, and isn't it so true? With every single client I have ever worked with that had food addiction, they too have had an unmet need or emotional imbalance in their lives. Most times these emotions could be traced back to core experiences or relationships that were traumatic or life altering. However, sometimes the emotions were simply job dissatisfaction, concern over money, lack of physical activity, etc. Once these emotions are dealt with properly, food can take a secondary role in our daily priorities. In my experience, until the emotions hidden beneath the surface can be addressed, food addiction will continue to be a struggle despite our efforts.

Thus, the next step in addressing food addiction is uncovering, experiencing, and properly addressing the emotional concerns that may be hiding or that we have tried to lock away. You may already know exactly what I am talking about and know what is causing the issue but may be afraid to address it. Or, you may be more like me, who had no idea what was causing the problem but recognized that my relationship with food was unhealthy. Either way, it is important to dig deep to discover what you are really feeling. You want to ask yourself, "what am I missing in my life that I am trying to replace with food?" Some of the best ways to explore this question is talking with a spouse, or friend; spending time alone with your thoughts meditating upon your feelings; journaling; or praying.

As we seek to find the problem and acknowledge its existence, it immediately begins to have less power over us. We can begin a plan of action or determine what steps we may need to take to fill that void within us so that we can heal. One of the tools used to help determine where the issue lies is a simple life satisfaction evaluation. Each of the categories should be rated on a scale of 1-10, 1 being extremely unsatisfied and 10 being satisfied. If you find a weak link, you will know where to begin your work! You may come back to this evaluation as often as needed to continue to

uncover emotions that may be plaguing you. Below is
an example.

Life Satisfaction Evaluation

Category	Rating
Overall Joy	
Spirituality	
Social Life	
Relationships	
Home Environment	
Education	
Career	
Finances	
Physical Activity	
Physical Health	
Home Cooking	
Creativity	

Gut Brain Connection

What many people don't know is that the brain and the digestive system are very closely linked. The gut is quite often referred to as our "second brain." The two organs are connected both physically and biochemically in a number of different ways.

The nervous system is the first link. Your gut contains approximately 500 million neurons.[97] These neurons send direct communication to the brain through the nervous system. The vagus nerve is one of the most predominant parts of your nervous system. It runs throughout your entire body and is the largest physical connection between the gut and brain. The vagus nerve is the only nerve in the body that originates from the brain stem and sends signals in both directions.[98] Interestingly, one study found that those with IBS and IBD also had probable vagus nerve dysfunction.[99]

The nervous system connection with the brain is strong in many other ways as well. For instance, within your nervous system, you have "nervous energy." Some also refer to this as "life force" or "life energy." The energy that moves exclusively through the nervous system is paramount for good health. However, this nervous energy can only be expended one of two ways. It can either be used to process emotions, or it can be used in digestion of difficult and processed foods.

Many will notice that when an emotional event occurs, they immediately reach for the so-called "comfort" foods. As you read in my story, I immediately went for my comfort foods after the big emotional and stressful events. Those who subconsciously do not want to deal with stress or emotions quite frequently overeat or eat bad foods to numb the pain. But the opposite is true as well. When we stop eating difficult to digest foods, emotions surface and it's quite a tender and vulnerable process. It's a double-edged sword, but eating clean is key to clearing out that toxic nerve energy and clearing the body and mind of these behaviors.

Additionally, our gut and brain are connected through gut microbes. Trillions of these microbes exist in your gut, and many of them are responsible for producing chemicals that impact your brain.[100] The short-chain fatty acids that are created in the gut can have a direct impact on your mental health and happiness. The healthier your gut microbiome is, the healthier the brain.

The final gut-brain connection worth mentioning is neurotransmitters. Neurotransmitters are produced in the brain, and they control our feelings and emotions. Our gut is responsible for creating many neurotransmitters as well. For instance, 90% of the serotonin in our body (responsible for our internal clock, sleep, and happiness) is created in our gut.[101] Our gut is also responsible for creating gamma-aminobutyric acid (GABA), which controls feelings of fear and anxiety.[102] These neurotransmitters are essential to our mental health and physical well-being. Studies have indicated that food choices dramatically impact the production of these neurotransmitters.[103]

These connections are incredibly important to note when we are dealing with food addiction. They indicate that the state of our gut directly impacts the state of our brain. If we are to overcome food addiction, we surely need both in good working order. Without the gut being healthy, the brain will never be able to function at an optimal level. And with a half functioning brain, your chances of overcoming addiction are greatly diminished. In order to take advantage of this connection, it is important to do everything possible to fortify the gut. Thus, by following the Crohn's Reversal Diet, you will be able to strengthen the gut which will enable you to more easily overcome food addiction naturally, as your brain is able to perform its proper functions.

Seek Professional Help

Recognizing the feelings behind why you are addicted to food may be difficult, but even more difficult is changing and reversing the behavior. After you have a firm idea of what is stopping your progress, it is time to spring into action. For many of my clients, simple exercises are not enough, and they need to enlist a professional to help them. There is nothing to be ashamed of by asking for help! These professionals have been trained and have the tools necessary to help our struggling brain to make the leap that is essential for our well-being.

Some people choose to see a personal counselor. For those that may not have a trusted friend or family member to talk openly with, this is a wonderful option. This can help one to express their feelings, seek advice, do specific exercises and have accountability as they work on their food addiction concerns.

I have also seen a 12-step program be very effective for many people. These programs help to work through these issues while you have support. Many don't realize there are entire organizations dedicated to the issue, such as Overeaters Anonymous (OA) or Food Addicts in Recovery Anonymous (FA). These are dedicated programs with trained professionals who can help you in your journey to overcome food addiction. Finding support in your journey to overcome your addiction is an imperative step.

Set Clear Boundaries

I found that setting clear limits for myself was also helpful. I sat down and made a list with three columns. On the left I wrote down foods that I promised to never eat again. Foods like meat, dairy, eggs, sugar, junk food, etc. In the middle, I made a list of foods that I can have in small doses on occasion like cold-pressed oil, ancient grain flours, carob or cacao, salt, etc. On the right I made a list of all of my favorite foods that I can eat unlimited amounts of. Since I made that list, I have never once indulged in the foods I committed not to eat again. I made a promise with myself and set clear boundaries that those items were always off limits. Additionally, I set clear guidelines for the "occasional" foods on the right. For instance, I committed to use oil no more than once a month, or flour products twice a month. After posting these goals on the fridge where I could refer back to them often, I checked in with my husband and God to give an account of how I was doing.

In addition to organizing and making the list, it is also helpful to have a plan. I find that in my own life, when I start my day with no plan for what I will make or what I will do, I end up snacking, making desserts, or eating out much more frequently. It is helpful to make a weekly meal plan. It can be simple and straightforward. Here is an example:

Monday
Breakfast: Smoothie
Lunch: Salad
Dinner: Buckwheat bowl
Snacks: Edamame beans and apples

It doesn't need to be specific or in depth if you don't want it to be. Just have a basic plan and idea of what you will eat that day. If you have a list and already have a plan you are more likely to stick with the plan and not give way to cravings or addictions. Be flexible with it, as you can change things whenever needed. Just have an outline that will keep you on track when the food addiction starts to rear its ugly head.

Although each of these steps has proven helpful for myself and many others that I have worked with, I cannot guarantee that you will overcome food addiction. It is a nasty beast, and I've had clients yell, swear, and start crying on the phone as we developed a plan to overcome these addictive foods. What I can say is that no harm will come from exploring these options. It should also be noted that depending on the depth of the food addiction, you may need to take care of the addiction before you can address the IBD or IBS symptoms. Only you will know which one you need to address first, but I don't recommend doing both at the same time.

To recap:

- Eat healthy foods and avoid all addictive foods
- Remember "food is fuel" and let each bite count
- Try to find the emotional cause of the food addiction and remedy it
- You have nervous energy that can only go to 1 of 2 things; digesting food or processing emotions
  - Stay clear of habit-forming or addictive foods
  - Eat real and unprocessed foods and eat until you are satiated
- Make a 3-column list and set clear limits for yourself on what you won't do, what you will occasionally do, and what you will often do
- Set boundaries and always have a plan

Chapter Five

More Stories

Though it is exciting to share, my story of healing was only the beginning of my journey. When I first got better, word spread among family and friends. People started coming to me to ask for help and advice, but I didn't really feel qualified to teach other people about health just yet. However, I was excited to share what I did know, even though it wasn't always met with appreciation. My circle quickly grew and before I knew it, I had a group of "clients" who were eager to learn. Because I was relatively new at this, I started teaching weekly lessons for free. Those weekly lessons quickly expanded and pretty soon, someone wanted one-on-one lessons. I would meet weekly with her, and within a few weeks I had another client. I hadn't done a shred of advertising, but people kept coming! Pretty soon, I had a great number of people asking for help, all from word of mouth. The more people that came, the better I became as a mentor, teacher, and aide. Since that time, I have educated thousands across the world on reversing chronic health conditions.

I have worked to educate people about nutrition and diet who have had every disease you can imagine—from thyroid disorders to diabetes to Crohn's disease and heart disease. I firmly believe, as Dr. John R. Christopher once stated, "there are no incurable diseases, only incurable people." Anyone who wants to get better truly can, and the power to act is within themselves. I've selected a few of my favorite stories to share with you in hopes that you will gain greater confidence that you too can overcome whatever obstacles lie in your path.

Why Haven't I Heard This Before?

Before we get to some of these stories, I want to answer a question you may have right now: "Cassidy, with all of this research and data available, why have I not heard of this until now?" To answer this complex question, I'll turn your attention to an experience I had in early 2019.

After I got well, I vowed that I would dedicate my life to helping others to receive the same miracle of healing that I had enjoyed. Word of my research spread quickly, and I had numerous invitations for speaking engagements. This was exciting to me, and these events were usually met with awe and gratitude. On one particular occasion, however, my message was met with what seemed to be major pushback.

I had been invited to speak at an event for a prominent IBD support group, with the organizers knowing full well (I assumed) that my whole expertise was in the field of diet and nutrition. I was excited to be sharing the latest studies on nutrition with the fellow Crohn's and colitis sufferers to give them hope for their future. I eagerly sent my presentation slides to the event organizers ahead of time for approval. That's when things got awkward.

The organizers called me on the phone and asked me to delete all the slides that shared research about diet reversing Crohn's and colitis. I was a bit caught off guard because I thought they would be excited about this. My contact then proceeded to tell me that they "wanted to focus their attention on pharmaceuticals since they were the ones funding the organization and the event." My jaw nearly dropped to the floor! Was this organization really willing to hide or ignore valuable information about the ability to obtain remission and healing because of money? In retrospect, I may have been a bit naive.

I confidently reasserted my position that the research I was to present was solid, and that I would be happy to send more research that was outside the scope of my presentation. The excuse then became that their scientists didn't have time to cross-vet the studies to make sure that the information wouldn't harm any of the IBD patients that would be in attendance, even though I was only sharing my experience and story backed up with research. After this, she never called me back but later emailed saying that diet changes were "not in alignment with the organization's current stance on the role that diet and nutrition play in the treatment of IBD." She then gave me an ultimatum of either not talking about diet in my presentation (which was 97% of the presentation) or not coming at all. I wasn't about to shy away from what I knew to be true, so I didn't go. Interestingly enough, a client who attended the event later informed me that they prepared a 45-minute presentation dedicated to spreading the anti-scientific claim that there is nothing that can be done for IBD in terms of diet and that dietary changes cannot help those who suffer from IBD. Ironically, the meeting ended with a solicitation for donations to help find a cure for Crohn's disease. Perhaps even more ironic was that I had worked with the event organizers to have a plant-based chef provide foods that would be easy on digestion for those with Crohn's and colitis. My client later informed me that one person even remarked that they felt so good after having the food, whereas they usually would be in pain.

This is the sad reality that we live in! I tell this story, not to point fingers at people who might disagree, but to shine a light on the current system of dealing with Crohn's, colitis, and other autoimmune diseases. When treatment and "cure" research are funded by pharmaceutical companies, there is no motivation to study the impact of dietary and lifestyle changes. It is unfortunate that even when there is groundbreaking research showing that diet changes can reverse chronic disease, most in the medical community hardly bat an eye. No one would make money if people were told to eat the foods from their gardens. Truly, when Hippocrates said to "let thy food be thy medicine," he probably wasn't thinking about the economics of it all.

Just because modern medicine hasn't found a cure for IBD, that doesn't mean there isn't hope. My goal in this chapter is to highlight a few healing journeys from people that, in the depths of despair, found hope– people who never thought they could get better but found healing through the IBD Reversal Diet. So, no, this is not some wacky plan. Many people have traversed a path similar to the one I took and found greater health as a result.

Amanda's Story

When Amanda was 16 years old, she started having severe digestive issues. It wasn't until she was 21 that she received the official diagnosis of Crohn's disease. She was heartbroken and didn't know where to start. She began taking the medications, but nothing changed. Four years later, at the young age of 25, Amanda went to the doctor's office with more problems. It was there that she was diagnosed with colon cancer. "I was in a state of complete shock," she said. Cancer at age 25 was not in the plan for Amanda. It was highly traumatic, and she didn't know who to turn to for help. Her doctors put her on more medications than she could count, and she was pumped full of pills for years, not understanding the effects it would have on her health. Her hair started falling out, she was exhausted, she was experiencing depression, and she had many other complications.

One day, she had a terrifying incident that changed everything. She started having extreme stabbing pain in her abdomen, and she couldn't breathe. They rushed her to the ER but no answers could be found. Her doctors simply brushed off the experience and told her diet and lifestyle had nothing to do with her health problems. That's when she decided it was time for a change. She was ready to take charge of her future, so she contacted me.

Amanda started on the IBD Reversal Diet, and to say she was skeptical would be an understatement. She had done years of study herself and questioned the methods that seemed so contrary to what she had learned from others. She said, "I would eat good stuff and then have a cheat meal, and it would immediately bring back all the pain. Then I was like, 'Let me stop messing around and let's do this. I have nothing to lose.'" It was often hard for her to stay motivated and restrict the foods she loved, but she decided to give it a shot. It was then that everything started to fall into place for her.

Within days of deciding to stick with it, she started sleeping better, she had improved bowel movements, her skin cleared up, she lost weight, and she even went off her medications. When she was taking her medications, she reported that she still had to nap every day just to make it through. Within a few weeks of focusing on foods, however, she no longer needed a nap and found that she had more energy than ever before. Within a few months, all of her symptoms were gone. To this day Amanda is both cancer free and Crohn's free! When she went to her doctor, he told her that she had previously had the worst case of IBD he had ever seen and was so astonished at her clear results that he ordered more tests just to confirm because it was so unbelievable. After those additional tests came back clear, he ordered her to continue coming in periodically to be monitored because he was shocked that a case that bad could be remedied. She said, "I am definitely the healthiest I have ever been–not only from a superficial standpoint, but my hair is thicker, my skin is softer, my joints don't hurt. I've lost weight and can maintain a balanced weight. From an internal perspective, my energy is the best it's ever been. I don't need naps to make it throughout the day. I don't ever feel like I am sad or depressed. All of that combined has brought me to my best self. There is no doctor or pill that could have gotten me to this point."

Taleah's Story

With good overall health, Taleah had never paid much attention to her diet. She had lived a pretty pain-free life until early 2019. Just after the holiday season, she had a Gall-bladder attack that sent her on a search for answers. As these episodes increased she didn't know what to do, and started searching for a path to healing.

This led Taleah to a big change in diet. When we started working together, she was overwhelmed and ready to try anything. We used a modified IBD Reversal Diet to cleanse her liver and gallbladder. Undergoing a 12-week cleanse was difficult, but rewarding. She said, "Though I wasn't perfect at maintaining the temporary diet restrictions, it still helped immensely!" By using healing foods, lifestyle changes, and herbs, she was able to clear out her body and see incredible improvements in her symptoms. "I am happy to say that my body felt so much better! I felt more balanced, more calm in my digestive system, more energy. But the best thing is that I haven't had a severe shoulder pain episode since last summer," she explained. She truly believes that she was able to avoid having her gallbladder removed and a subsequent lifetime of complications because of the changes that she made. She believes that, "Food is a gift–a fuel to sustain our bodies, and medicine to heal it and strengthen it."

Michael's Story

Michael was a healthy boy, aside from the occasional stomach ache after a meal. He was a budding cross-country star at his high school and had a great love for the outdoors. At age 17, his trajectory in life was dramatically altered. It began when, after cross-country races, Michael found himself dealing with excruciating stomach pains. It got so bad that he went to the doctor, and after a series of tests and the dreaded colonoscopy, he was diagnosed with ulcerative colitis. That diagnosis rocked his world, and things started getting worse. Before long, he had to quit cross-country. He even had to drop out of school entirely. He would spend his whole day lying on the couch, unable to move or perform basic functions. Michael couldn't even get up without having to take Zofran. The pain was unbearable every single day. "The medication helped a little, but it caused so many other side effects," he said. By this time, his weight had dropped to just over 100 pounds, even though he was 6'4". Unsure if he could survive much longer in this condition, his mom reached out to me in desperation.

When he began working with me, he immediately started a cleanse to get the right nutrients for his body. It was a difficult road for him as a teenage boy. Michael recounted, "I noticed immediate relief the first day, my stomach pain was completely gone. But then it came back for a few weeks while I cleansed, and I haven't had stomach pain since. Once I got off the medication, the rest of the symptoms went away." Though he was anxious to put healthy weight back on, it took a few weeks to see results. Within a few months, though, he weighed in at a healthy 132, a number he previously thought would be impossible to see.

But that wasn't all. He excitedly said, "I was able to do cross-country again. I started going to school again. I could go on a hike and rock climb. Pretty much everything I couldn't do before I can now." His mom called in tears one day saying, "Every time I think about where he's been and what you've done so far to help him, I'm brought to tears and am so full of gratitude."

Rachel's Story

In 2010, Rachel was diagnosed with severe Crohn's disease. For years, she struggled in pain to find any kind of relief. She tried every medication on the market, and each one either didn't help at all or exacerbated her problems. She was desperate for answers and willing to try anything to get relief. The doctors recommended a colostomy, and she readily accepted, hoping this would be the long-awaited answer. After the first surgery didn't produce the desired results, she underwent five additional surgeries in hopes of finding healing. However, none of these were successful, either. In fact, after these painful operations, she was worse than ever. She grew more and more upset and wondered if she would ever have hope for a normal life.

She was so disillusioned with the medical route that she started to look for more natural remedies. Each new doctor or specialist that she found had different answers for her, yet none of them seemed to work. She tried every diet in the book and still felt the same. It wasn't until she became pregnant with her second child that things hit rock bottom. She said, "I went into an emergency delivery because my body was shutting down, and we wanted to save the baby and me. After having the baby, I was flat in bed. I couldn't even take care of my two precious boys. I couldn't even be present in my lifelong dream of being a mother, and it was more than I could bear." Luckily for Rachel, that was the exact moment that our paths crossed.

When we started the IBD Reversal Diet, things were rocky. In addition to her Crohn's-specific symptoms, she had abscesses and fistulas from the surgery and the colostomy bag. She went through some incredible days and some extremely difficult days. Her body had gone through so much in such a short time, and the cleansing process was difficult for her. But even during the cleanse, she felt better than she had her entire life. She said, "My energy started to come back and my pain started to go away. I can't even explain how amazing it was to watch my body heal. It took me about six months to feel like I was healed. But what is six months when I've been in so much pain for *ten years*?! I now believe that food can heal anybody and any health condition. You just have to know what foods are good for you and what foods hurt your body. It's healed my gut, it helped my husband, and it's healed my baby's eczema."

Phillip's Story

When Phillip was diagnosed with diabetes, he was beside himself. He faithfully followed his doctor's orders and ate a low carb diet for many years. He was taught that carbs were the enemy and would cause more issues, so he avoided them like the plague for nearly 10 years. He says that he tried every diet he could find: "I even had some short-term success, but was never able to stay with it over the long-term."

Additionally, Phillip took a handful of medications for years as he tried to manage his diabetes the conventional way. In early 2020, Philip landed in the hospital with a blood sugar reading of over 500! After this scary experience, he knew it was time for a big change and reached out to me. Even though my specialty is with IBD, I taught him about the principles in this book because they work! He began eating the right diet, using herbs, and changing up a number of other small things. Within just a few weeks sticking to the plan, he lost over 35 lbs and went off all of his medications. "I can't tell you how great I feel. I am now off of all of my diabetic medicine, usually waking up with a blood glucose reading of 85 or 90," he once told me. Last time we spoke, he told me he took several walks a day just because he had so much energy. He told me that he wanted to shout it from the rooftops and let people know that diet is the answer everyone is looking for. There is a path to healing, and it's with food.

Ashley's Story

Ashley suffered for over 10 years, searching for answers to her severe abdominal pain and digestive issues. She endured every test, doctors visit, and colonoscopy necessary to get to the bottom of her growing list of health concerns. Throughout her life, even though she was in severe pain, she was a happy, adventurous, and energetic girl. But, now she was at her lowest, experiencing extreme fatigue, anxiety, and depression along with her debilitating intestinal problems. She worked with countless doctors, naturopaths, and other experts to find an answer. After a decade of no answers, she was finally diagnosed with severe Crohn's disease. "That day was the single most heartbreaking, gut-wrenching, and stressful day of my life," she recounted. Her doctors told her that she would never again be able to eat any nuts, seeds, beans, legumes, raw fruits, raw vegetables, onion, garlic, spicy foods, and grains. They also told her that she would need to be on medication for the rest of her life, with no chances of getting off and that she would likely be hospitalized multiple times. She was heartbroken, scared, and hopeless.

She did as she was told but didn't see any results. She was still feeling horribly sick and the infusions weren't helping, plus they were extremely expensive. Additionally, all of this treatment gave her intense arthritis that made many activities unbearable. She wondered how she could spend the rest of her life in pain and continually getting worse. After a year of these failed methods she says, "all of my prayers were answered after I found Cassidy through a lucky series of events on Instagram where a girl had reached out to me and told me about Cassidy who had turned her life back around through diet."

I started meeting with Ashley immediately, but It wasn't all fun and games. She says, "There is no denying that beginning this diet was one of the hardest things I've ever done–I was the biggest foodie I know and to suddenly go to eating three meals a day that mostly consisted of rice and potatoes seemed like torture." But she persevered. Though it was tough work, she stayed strict on the diet and almost immediately began seeing improvements. Her inflammation decreased, and very soon she stopped taking naps. Before long, she was able to hike for miles with no problem, something that was previously impossible. "For the first time in years I actually started to feel like myself again–physically, mentally, and emotionally," she later told me. Though she had a few slip-ups along the way, she has done an amazing job at staying true to the IBD Reversal Diet. When I asked Ashley to elaborate on how she felt after healing herself with this diet she said, "At this point I can honestly say that I feel better than I have felt in over 10 years, and I still cry on a regular basis because I just feel so thankful for where I am now compared to where I was before.

I'm happier than I've ever been; I have more energy than I've ever had; my body is completely pain free; I have gained all the weight that I lost back; and eating this diet feels like the biggest reward to me. Every single person that has been in my life through this journey continuously comments on how happy and healthy I look these days, and it never gets old hearing it."

Common Themes

Though each person's story is different, there are a few common themes. The first is that for many people, they weren't willing to make the necessary changes until things looked very dire. This was certainly the case for me. I wasn't willing to make difficult and seemingly drastic changes until I felt like there were no other options. As humans, we want to move along the path of least resistance. This is ironic when it comes to our health because if we would just make the necessary changes, we would have greater health and more personal freedom.

Another common thread in all of these stories (and others) is that our bodies are amazing and know what to do to make us well. We just need to provide them with the right stuff. Truly, food has the power to heal. When we stop putting the harmful substances in our bodies and start putting the right things in, our bodies can spring into action to start the healing process. It saddens me when I hear that people don't believe we can become well with what nature has provided. Even though many medical professionals are now realizing and studying the power of everyday foods, a majority of doctors and health practitioners, unfortunately, have a hard time accepting this knowledge.

The last common theme in these stories is that despite the varying circumstances, change is possible! Yes, you can physically change! All too often I see people who believe that they are their disease or condition. When presented with information that could change their condition and their life, they play the victim card stating that there is nothing you can do for [insert condition], and they just have to suffer for the rest of their life. What a sad perspective! I often have to remind myself that if someone doesn't want to change for the better, their choice needs to be respected. However, for me and for many others, it has been so empowering to realize that we don't have to be stuck with pain and suffering for the rest of our lives. We are not our diseases. We can overcome our health challenges to lead healthy and happy lives.

I used to think that the greatest measure of success for my life was how many trophies, awards, or accolades I could win. I have now come to believe that true success comes from helping to relieve someone else's burden. And if you have Crohn's disease or ulcerative colitis, you *know* just how much of a burden it can be. There aren't many things that bring me greater joy than hearing about someone's healing journey. I am so grateful that I have been able to witness and be a small part of many.

Chapter Six

Frequently Asked Questions

Beginning the IBD Reversal Diet may seem overwhelming at first, and many people come to me with a laundry list of questions. Below, I have compiled the most frequently asked questions that I receive.

What about fiber?

An estimated 97 percent of the population is fiber deficient, yet fiber is one of the most important nutrients for our bodies.[104] It has been proven to reduce the risk of diabetes, heart disease (including high cholesterol, blood pressure, and blood sugars), obesity, and various cancers.[105] Despite all of this, many have been told that fiber is the enemy for a number of ailments, including IBD and IBS. This, however, couldn't be further from the truth. In fact, a 19 study meta-analysis concluded that IBD patients who ate diets that were high in animal fats had significantly worse symptoms.[106] The analysis also found that diets high in fiber from fruits and vegetables had lower risk of IBD and IBS symptoms. But this isn't all. Another important study concluded that avoiding fiber is associated with a 60 percent increased risk of IBD flares over a 6-month period.[107]

Many studies back up these claims, and the ultimate consensus is that a high fiber diet is one of the most effective tools in treating IBD, often leading to permanent remission.[108] I have seen this happen in my own life and in the lives of others. Though it is wise to add fiber in gradually so the system doesn't become overloaded all at once, it is one of the best sources of nutrition and healing that we have.

How long does it take to heal?

The healing timeline depends entirely upon the person. I've worked with people who have said they felt better immediately, and I've worked with others who took nearly six months. You have to remember that there are many factors to consider like genetics, toxic build up, previous surgeries, emotional balance, etc. I wish it was a cookie cutter experience for people to heal from these difficult diseases, but it's not that simple. The key, however, is to not be discouraged when it's not happening in the timeline you had imagined. There are many ways to cleanse, so if one isn't working, it doesn't mean you should give up. Again, I am convinced that there are no incurable diseases, only incurable people. As long as you aren't an incurable person, healing will come!

What other substances should I avoid?

I have found that avoiding products such as sodas, energy drinks, alcohol, coffee, all non-herbal teas, and other similar products is very helpful to healing. These enervating substances slow the healing process and can cause additional complications. Coffee, for instance, promotes acid reflux and gastroesophageal reflux.[109] Alcohol dramatically increases symptoms for both IBD and IBS patients.[110] Wine and soft drinks are also closely related to worsened symptoms of IBD.[111] Of course, all illicit drugs should be avoided whenever possible, as these are inflammatory and are associated with many health risks. Unfortunately, many people are addicted to these kinds of substances and products. Once you remove them for a couple of weeks, you can really see the difference. When you try to reintroduce them, you'll notice that they do not make your body feel good.

For those that suffer from IBD or IBS, I have seen almonds cause significant issues for a number of people. Though there is no data specifically linking almonds with IBS, there is some data to suggest that excess sulfur and sulfate dramatically worsen symptoms.[112] Since almonds are high in sulfur, this could possibly be the connection.[113] The evidence is spotty, but many of my clients have seen that removing almonds helps their digestion greatly.

Can you get enough protein without meat?

A protein is a combination of 20 or 22 amino acids, depending on who you ask.[114] Some of these amino acids are produced naturally in the body, so we don't have to worry about them. The remaining 9 amino acids are what we call "essential," which means our body does not naturally produce them, and they must, therefore, be obtained from food. The good news is that these amino acids all originate in the dirt and in plant foods![115] That means the best way to get these amino acids is from plants. Many are shocked to find that there is virtually no such thing as protein deficiency–just the opposite is true. A recent study found that a high animal protein intake is associated with a 75 percent increased risk in overall mortality and a 400 percent increase in cancer.[116] In essence, it's more likely that you can have *too much* protein rather than too little.

Surprisingly, our best source of protein comes from plants. When you think about it, where do the animals that humans eat get their protein? From plants! Why not just cut out the middle-man and go straight to the source of the nutrients? I don't think I've ever heard of a cow or a gorilla being protein deficient because they didn't eat enough meat. It is also important to note that studies indicate our bodies need only about 10 percent of our daily caloric intake from protein.[117] That means the average 150 lb. person only needs about 50 grams of protein per day, even for bodybuilders.[118]

Furthermore, overconsumption of protein, in particular animal protein, is linked to autoimmune diseases such as diabetes, kidney disease, MS, IBS, and Lyme disease.[119] One study found a significantly increased risk of developing diabetes on a high animal protein diet.[120] Another study found a 60 percent *increased* risk of heart disease on an animal protein diet and a 40 percent *decreased* risk on a diet of plant-based proteins.[121] These studies and many others indicate that plant sources are not only a superior form of protein but they lead to significantly improved health outcomes. From a scholastic perspective, the data is overwhelming.

Can you get enough calcium without dairy?

When it comes to dairy, I often find that it is best to take a step back and look at the bigger picture. Dairy products come from the milk from a cow. And that milk is the perfect food . . . for a baby cow! Cow's milk was designed for a cow, and as such it's filled with everything necessary to turn a small calf into a 500-pound beast. Mother's milk–the perfect food for a baby human–is significantly different from the milk of a cow. This is because humans and cows are genetically very different. If we turned the tables and fed human milk to a baby calf, the baby calf wouldn't get the proper nutrition it needs to grow into a healthy, full grown cow.

The big concern with eliminating dairy for many people is that they won't get enough calcium in their diet, eventually leading to weak bones, osteoporosis, etc. But when it comes to calcium, can we get enough without dairy? And can we still have strong bones without dairy? The answers to these questions are yes, absolutely! For many years in western society we have been sold a narrative that humans need cow's milk in order to develop properly and have strong bones, but this couldn't be further from the truth. While it is true that milk contains a good amount of calcium, many plant foods have just as much. Additionally, the absorption rate of calcium by the body (which is what really matters) from many plant foods is as good or better than that of milk. For example, the absorption rate of kale is nearly 60 percent while the absorption rate of milk is only 32 percent.[122] Additionally, studies have not been able to show that an increased intake of calcium or milk will lead to a decreased risk of bone fracture.[123]

I've tried a plant based diet and it didn't work. How is this different?

I hear this one a lot! The IBD Reversal Diet is more than just eating plants and calling it a day. After the intestines have undergone so much stress and disease, even very healing foods that are incredible for us, like spinach and broccoli, can not be tolerated at first. Varying genetics, diets, stressors, medical history, etc. can make a one-size-fits-all approach difficult. But understanding the basic principles and parameters for healing are sure to help even the most difficult of diseases. Following the IBD Reversal Diet or a similar cleansing protocol is the first step for ANY disease, not just Crohn's and ulcerative colitis.

Many may have tried a generic plant based diet before, but did they detox first? Were they allergic to the pesticides being used on the fruit? Were there emotional stressors that overpowered food choices? There are so many considerations when looking at disease! The small nuances of the diet matter, and perhaps with the knowledge in this book, you will be empowered to give it another go.

Why don't doctors teach this?

A lot of this information can be hard to take in and believe, because it is not often talked about in the mainstream. Many people believe that if their doctor doesn't preach it, that must mean it's not true. However, many doctors do know and have published research on many of the cited claims. The question on everyone's mind is: "So why don't a majority of doctors know or teach this?" I truly believe that a good number of doctors really care about their patients and only want what they believe is best for them. However, there are a couple of variables to keep in mind that might not be so obvious.

First of all, research has shown that doctors in general don't receive very much instruction in medical school on the subject of nutrition. One study from 2014 showed that most medical schools fall far short of the recommended amount of nutrition instruction.[124] The study also showed that an overwhelming majority of instructors surveyed at these schools believed that the amount of nutrition education in the curriculum was inadequate. There usually aren't classes solely dedicated to nutrition. The nutritional education is usually diluted as a section of a physiology or biology class. This lack of nutrition knowledge can even be confirmed by test scores. One study took a group of medical professionals and tested their knowledge on diet and nutrition among other topics. The average score among the practicing doctor group was 62 percent.[125] That's a failing grade! Perhaps this helps explain why many physicians feel unprepared or inadequate to provide patients with dietary advice.[126]

The next thing to consider is "where is the money?" We don't often hear about the vegetable industry being indicted on fraud, corruption, and conspiracy, but there is one industry that is notorious for such things: pharmaceuticals.[127] Indeed, the U.S. pharmaceutical market is nearly a half-trillion dollar industry.[128] And Big Pharma has spent some big bucks on making sure it keeps going up. For years it has been well known that pharmaceutical companies pour large sums of money into influencing medical schools, often creating conflicts of interest.[129] If fruits and vegetables can help with certain conditions more effectively and for less money than a drug, those with a pill to sell you wouldn't want that knowledge to be taught. This influence from Big Pharma doesn't just stop in medical school, however. A professor from UCLA researched the influence of pharmaceutical companies on doctors and found that the companies "are spending something like double the amount that they spend on research and development [of new drugs] on marketing to doctors."[130] Pharma is also usually one of the top spenders when it comes to contributing to political campaigns and to lobbying Congress. In 2019, for example, total lobbying expenditures by the pharmaceutical industry equalled $29,301,000.[131] In short, there's a lot of money to be made from pharmaceuticals, but I have yet to meet someone who has become rich from farming and selling broccoli or kale.

In my opinion, doctors have a lot to handle and are often very knowledgeable and skilled when it comes to drugs and medications; their realm simply isn't nutrition. I'm not a doctor and can't even fathom all the amount of time it takes in medical school to receive and master that kind of training. My specialty is food, which has been around much longer than our modern drugs and doesn't require as intensive of study. There is a place for medication and there is a place for food.

Does the IBD Reversal Diet help with other diseases?

Yes, yes and yes! The principles behind each step are the same principles I have used for years in helping others. Though each personal situation may require slight adjustments, the overall concept of detoxifying, building the gut, using herbs, avoiding animal foods, and focusing on real, whole plant foods is the same premise used by thousands across the world to heal from all sorts of diseases.

We live in a world that has largely forgotten that food is fuel (and medicine) for our bodies, and nature knows how to make the foods that will do us the most good. What God has designed, man has perverted by hijacking our taste buds in the name of profit. When we get back to the real, simple, and healthy foods, we will be able to find healing.

Will I experience detox symptoms when I start?

When I started healing, I experienced some intense symptoms! Even though I felt better than I had previously, I experienced a runny nose, headache, soreness, and more. But this wasn't the worst of it. As I began eating healthier I became an emotional wreck. I was more emotional than I had ever been, and a lifetime of bottled-up feelings surfaced all at once. I would later learn that because nerve energy can only go to either difficult-to-digest foods or processing emotions, that was the first time all of my nerve energy had been centered on emotions. And boy, was it intense! I had never had to face some of these feelings and memories before, and that was a side effect I didn't anticipate from cleansing. I would later learn that this is the case for many who undergo such shifts in diet. It was something for which I was ill prepared.

Though this was the case for me, this is not the case with every person I work with. Some of my clients report feeling great and having no complications, and others report feeling very lethargic and sick for a short time in the beginning. What can we expect after allowing toxic substances into our systems for so many years?

Are there other factors that contribute to IBD I should be aware of?

Many autoimmune diseases are directly linked to diet. Thousands of studies show that diet is a primary cause of nearly every disease from diabetes, heart diseases, and thyroid disorders, to multiple sclerosis, arthritis, and more.[132] IBD has recently been classified as a lifestyle disease. Though microbial dysbiosis (aka diet) has been found to be the number one cause, there are a number of other lifestyle factors that contribute.[133] Aside from simply eating the right foods, one should consider eating small, frequent meals as opposed to three large meals in a day.[134]

Stress is thought to be one of the major contributors to Crohn's and Colitis.[135] I've seen great success with many clients as they either get rid of big stressors in their life or learned to handle them appropriately. Their conditions are greatly improved by implementing proper exercise, relaxation techniques, and sleep hygiene. I have seen a common theme among nearly all of my IBD clients: each one of them had emotional distress that contributed to their condition. Their symptoms flare up when they are exposed to those stressors.

Of course, there are many other considerations too, such as genetics, toxic exposure, relationships, etc. But in my experience, most autoimmune diseases can be reversed or greatly helped with diet.

Chapter Seven

Knowledge is Power

Real health takes work. I wish I could tell you that if you just do these four steps you'll be healed with minimal effort, but unfortunately that isn't the case. There is no magic bullet that can heal chronic disease. True healing often takes time, especially when the body has undergone years of malnutrition and abuse. In fact, despite feeling relief within days of beginning my IBD Reversal Diet, it took me months to fine tune my health and get everything where I wanted it to be. It took daily effort to keep on my health, and I had to use herbs daily for several months before I could produce three to four healthy bowel movements each day completely unassisted. Here I am years later with no symptoms of Crohn's disease as I eat a minimally processed, oil-free, whole food, plant based diet. And you can be, too!

Throughout any healing journey, it certainly isn't all sunshine and roses. Some days are more difficult than others. I've sat through sessions with clients who just cry in anguish, wondering if they can make it one more day on rice and potatoes. Conversely, I have also sat through meetings with clients who cried with joy because they were free and their symptoms had disappeared. Although certain principles can apply to everyone, I really do wish there was a one-size-fits-all for healing. Some people take a few weeks and others take a few months, but the key is to not give up. I had one client who worked hard for months on end trying every cleanse and herb we could think of. With considerable improvements, but still experiencing some symptoms, we had to work extra hard to get to the root of her issues. But, just as she experienced, healing does come, in its own due time. This IBD Reversal Diet has worked for so many people who have made the commitment and followed through, even if it took adjustments and time. So, don't give up. Even when you feel like giving up, keep pressing forward.

Although most clients see incredible healing using this diet, sometimes clients will follow this way of eating exactly and still have some lingering issues. Each time, these issues can usually be traced back to one of four things:

1. Not chewing your food
2. Drinking water with meals
3. Emotional imbalances
4. Underlying yeast overgrowth (candida)

I believe it's important to take a deeper look at each of these issues so that you can tackle them if you are feeling like there are still issues that are not clearing up.

Chewing Food

Properly masticating food is a highly underrated practice in today's fast paced world. In a hurry, we grab our meal and chow it down in the car, not stopping for one second to enjoy the flavors or allow salivary digestion to perform the function nature intended. Most people don't realize that digestion begins in the mouth. The enzymes contained in our saliva are one of the most important factors in breaking down our food and preparing it for the stomach. The more time our food spends in the mouth, the better. I often repeat this common phrase to my clients: "drink your foods and chew your drinks." That means when you take a bite, it should spend enough time in the mouth to become liquefied. After you think you have chewed enough, keep chewing! This process will save the intestinal tract from having to do the work later on in the digestive process. If you can ease the burden on the bowels by simply eating slowly and chewing thoroughly, it will be well worth the inconvenience.

The evidence for thorough mastication is all too convincing. Researchers discovered a drastic difference in the digestion of those that were fed through feeding tubes versus those who were able to properly chew their food.[136] The digestive process was greatly improved for those that chewed their food in any capacity via the autonomic nervous function in the digestive tract. Moreover, there has been a marked improvement in energy among those who properly chew their food.[137] But one of the greatest benefits in the medical literature is the improved absorption of the nutrients in food. One study indicated that there was significantly greater nutrient absorption from almonds that were chewed 40 times versus those that were only chewed 10 times.[138]

I have noticed a theme among my IBD clients: they are all hasty eaters who take only a few bites before swallowing. In some instances, simply correcting their eating habits is enough to give relief to their digestive tract. The best way to begin this habit is to eat meals with no distractions. Take time to eat sitting down where you can slowly eat each bite and focus on the food you have. Oftentimes being more mindful and cultivating an attitude of gratitude around eating can help. It can also be helpful to give yourself a quota in the beginning as you start to chew properly. For instance, tell yourself you must chew at least 15 seconds or 10 bites before swallowing. This can help retrain the muscles and get you on the right track.

However you do it, it is important to start now to chew your food and chew it well!

Drinking Water With Meals

Another poor habit that should be stopped is drinking water with meals. Many people are surprised to learn this habit can be quite harmful since it is common among nearly all people to drink copious amounts of water while eating. Yet, this simple practice can lead to severe gas, bloating, indigestion, and more. This is because our bodies secrete enzymes to break down the various foods we eat. These enzymes start in the saliva, as discussed previously, and are present throughout the entire digestive process up to excretion. When we drink water as we eat, the water dilutes the enzymes in our mouth and neutralizes the pH of our stomach acid. This prevents our food from beginning the breakdown process until it's far too late to salvage. Then we start to see digestive woes that aren't remedied, even from proper eating.

Most of my clients look at me in shock when I first invite them to stop drinking with meals. It is an extremely difficult habit to break, but one that is well worth the effort. When people stop drinking with meals, they aren't sure when to drink water. They get stressed out, and they stop drinking altogether until dehydration sets in. The proper times to drink water are 15-30 minutes before a meal or two hours after a meal. I have found that drinking a large water bottle when I first wake up in the morning and drinking a water bottle 15 minutes before each meal allows me to get my proper water intake in without depressing my digestion or interfering with my busy life.

Now, this begs the next question, how much water should a person be drinking? The answer varies from person to person, but I generally recommend a minimum of 90 ounces per day. The ideal water consumption is a gallon a day, and that is what I aim for, yet this may still be too much for some, so drink as much as you are able. It may take time to work up to the point where you can drink that much water in a day, so take it day by day and increase your intake incrementally until you are at the ideal spot. The benefits of water consumption are endless, so drink up!

Emotional Imbalances

As I have already discussed, this little hiccup is perhaps the least popular, but one of the most important. It is nigh impossible to obtain optimal health while in a chronically stressed or highly emotional state. Emotional imbalances can stem from an abusive or traumatic childhood, a single life-altering event, unhealthy relationships, mental instability, systemic brain dysfunction, current abuse, financial strain, and so much more. Sometimes even with the greatest care, our bodies need additional emotional aid to overcome the last hurdle on our road to wellness. I know from personal experience.

When I first made an overhaul of my life and began eating healthier, I felt like a million dollars! After a few months, however, I felt that I had plateaued. And while I was still healthier than I had ever been, there was something holding me back from the final ascent to health. I struggled for a long time until I recognized that I had been holding in a great deal of anxiety, fear, and hurt from experiences I'd had years ago. As my raw emotions surfaced, I worked hard to clear through the hurt and to heal. It took years before I felt like I was free from my mental anguish. Once I truly balanced my emotions, I was a new person when it came to my health. It was as though my emotional problems were physically manifesting themselves through dysfunction in my body. After working through the emotions, those bodily dysfunctions disappeared.

Underlying Yeast Overgrowth

One of the last things to look for (or one of the first) is possible yeast overgrowth in the stomach. Candida is a fungus that grows in the stomach. Normally, this fungus is harmless and aids in breaking down sugar and alcohol. However, when this fungus overtakes the stomach, it can be difficult to get rid of and can cause many lingering health issues.

The most common way to get an overgrowth of candida is by taking antibiotics. Antibiotics kill off all bacteria in the stomach except for candida. That means the candida has room to spread out while the good gut bacteria take time to repopulate. The candida grows even more when you eat sugars (carbohydrates) and alcohol. Some of the most common symptoms of a candida overgrowth include: tiredness and fatigue, oral thrush, bad breath, urinary tract infections, sinus infections, digestive issues, and more. In fact, some research actually suggests that high levels of candida can be a trigger for IBD.[139]

There are many ways that you can get rid of a candida overgrowth; some of these ways take longer than others and some are more effective than others. The fastest and most permanent way that I have seen to eliminate a candida overgrowth is to go on a 30-day, plant based, ketogenic diet (high fat, low carb) with a combination of herbs to kill off the candida. The next step is to repopulate the good gut flora with probiotic-rich, natural foods such as kimchi, sauerkraut, pickles, etc. This type of diet isn't necessarily a walk in the park, but I can attest that it's fast and it works.

Choose Your Hard

I realize that it's hard to make changes. However, as you consistently make different choices, this new lifestyle will become easier. It is hard work, but so is being sick. Always maintaining proximity to a toilet is hard. Getting a colonoscopy (or multiple) is hard. So choose your hard. In my opinion, saying no to a burger is hard, but keeling over all night in pain is harder. I truly believe food is not worth the cost of good health. Poor eating is a mortgage on your health, a payment which will come due in the form of illness, disease, and a potential early death. Is the momentary pleasure derived from our modern "food" worth our future? I don't believe it is; I've been on both sides.

I'll never forget that time in the doctor's office trying to stomach the thought that I might not be able to have children, and if I did, I might not be around for very long with them. That thought was devastating to me. One of my number one priorities in life was to be a mother, and I thought I had lost the chance.

That moment spurred me into action; I found a reason to get better. Now, here I am years later with two wonderful children who I can help make better choices than the ones I made. Each of us with chronic health problems needs to figure out our own reason to heal. I just hope and pray that many people will make a decision to change before the circumstances get dire. It is much easier to reverse disease when it is young. The more it progresses, the more difficult it is to tackle.

Healing is Possible

When I set out to write this book, I had little idea what it would turn into. I didn't realize how cathartic it would be to write and share my own story of healing. I didn't want to talk about my past and my former life and was reluctant to write about it. The pageant queen engulfed in a fake life is not who I am anymore, and I look back in dismay of who I used to be. At the encouragement of friends and family, however, I realized this was a story that needed to be shared. It seemed like I had it all, but I didn't have anything at all. I was sick and miserable. Most people I knew admired me and wanted to be me, but I didn't feel admirable and often wanted to be someone else. I was a food addict, a slave, and unhappy, but no one had any idea.

I was brought to the depths of humility as I suffered in agony each day. When I realized I had nowhere to go but up, I was able to rebuild a better foundation for my life and my physical body. I was in a dark place, and I found hope. As my health increased, so did my mental well-being. I no longer felt the need to seek attention and praise, and I was able to find joy in motherhood, family, and cultivating the earth. Those are things I honestly never thought I would care about before, but they have come to be my whole world.

There is a special place in my heart for every person out there suffering with IBD and IBS, who feels that there is no hope for them. I have been there and have felt that. I thought I was in for a long life of pain, medication, and suffering. I had no idea that healing was not only possible, but affordable and simple. In my darkest times, I felt so sad and alone. Sometimes I wondered how I could go on. Throughout my time as a natural health educator, I have met with hundreds of people from around the world who I can look in the eyes and empathize with. You are not alone. We are not alone.

Unfortunately, I didn't find a cure for Crohn's disease in the traditional sense of the word. I don't know of a pill that will instantaneously make digestive problems go away. But I did find knowledge, and that knowledge is powerful. When we let go of the fake foods and fake lifestyles and get back to eating and living simply, our bodies respond quickly. When you apply this knowledge in your own life, you can see miracles! I don't believe that good health should be complicated. In fact, it's when we complicate things that we get ourselves in trouble and in poor health.

If there is one thing that I want you to learn from my story it's that healing is possible! I was basically told that I was a lost cause, and there was no hope for me to live a normal, healthy life. Yet, here I stand, in permanent remission from Crohn's disease and all the other problems I had. If I can do it, anyone can do it.

Acknowledgements

This book would not have been possible without the tireless work and encouragement of my husband, Jordan. I had the world's best editors–Niki Reeder and Judy Shepherd–who helped prepare this book for the public eye. I am also grateful to my in-laws, Troy and Valerie Gundersen, for their selfless sacrifice and support to make this book possible. I was blessed with the best group of friends, family, and clients that encouraged me along the process–a group too big to name here! A big thank you to Carol-Aynn Knott, Lily Sparks, Iris Thieme, Paige Norton, Amanda Weaver, Sonja Nyman, Carol Lewis, and Erica Rivera for your feedback and help to make this book so much better. And finally I want to acknowledge each one of my clients who has taught me so much and helped me to find a path to healing that would bless so many lives.

Notes

1. "Autoimmune Disease," *DrFurman.com*, https://www.drfuhrman.com/get-started/health-concerns/6/autoimmune-disease

2. Amadeo, Kimberly, "Medical Bankruptcy and the Economy," *The Balance*, 19 November 2019, https://www.thebalance.com/medical-bankruptcy-statistics-4154729

3. Sambamoorthi, Usha et al. "Multiple chronic conditions and healthcare costs among adults." *Expert review of pharmacoeconomics & outcomes research* vol. 15,5 (2015):823-32.

4. Dahlhamer, James M. et al. "Prevalence of Inflammatory Bowel Disease Among Adults Aged ≥18 Years — United States, 2015," *Morbidity and Mortality Weekly Report,* 2016;65:1166–1169.

5. Chey, William D. et al. "Irritable bowel syndrome: a clinical review," *Journal of the American Medical Association,* 2015;313(9):949–958.

6. Lewis, James D. and Maria T. Abreu, "Diet as a Trigger or Therapy for Inflammatory Bowel Diseases," *Gastroenterology*, 2017 Feb;152(2):398-414.

7. "Definition & Facts of Kidney Stones in Children," *National Institute of Diabetes and Digestive and Kidney Diseases*, May 2017, https://www.niddk.nih.gov/health-information/urologic-diseases/kidney-stones-children/definition-facts#common.

8. Lewis, James D. and Maria T. Abreu, "Diet as a Trigger or Therapy for Inflammatory Bowel Diseases," *Gastroenterology*, 2017 Feb;152(2):398-414.

9. See *The Word of Wisdom: Hope, Healing, and the Destroying Angel,* Restoration Publishing, August 2020.

10. *The Facts About Inflammatory Bowel Diseases*, Crohn's and Colitis Foundation of America, November 2014, pp. 6-7.

11. Ibid.

12. "Inflammatory Bowel Disease (IBD) Patients Experience Invisible and Life-altering Burdens," *Health Union*, 3 May 2017, https://health-union.com/news/inflammatory-bowel-disease-patients-experience-invisible-and-life-altering-burdens/

13. "Toxics Release Inventory (TRI) Program," United States Environmental Protection Agency, https://www.epa.gov/toxics-release-inventory-tri-program/tri-listed-chemicals

14. Fellizar, Kristine, "7 Subtle Signs Of Toxin Overload In Your Body," *Bustle*, 17 October 2018.

15. Crinnion, Walter J., "The CDC fourth national report on human exposure to environmental chemicals: what it tells us about our toxic

burden and how it assist environmental medicine physicians," *Alternative Medicine Review*, July 2010, vol. 15(2):101-9.

16. Dórea, Jose G., "Persistent, bioaccumulative and toxic substances in fish: human health considerations," *Science of the Total Environment*, August 2008, vol. 400(1-3):93-114.
17. Reid, Gregor et al., "Potential uses of probiotics in clinical practice." *Clinical microbiology reviews*, 2003, vol. 16(4):658-72.
18. Stewart, WF et al., "Epidemiology of constipation (EPOC) study in the United States: relation of clinical subtypes to sociodemographic features," *American Journal of Gastroenterology*, 1999;94:3530-3540.
19. Birt, Diane F. et al., "Resistant Starch: Promise for Improving Human Health," *Advances in Nutrition*, November 2013, vol. 4(6):587–601.
20. "Colitis (Severe), Inflammatory Bowel Disease, Ulcerative Colitis, Crohn's Disease," *DrMcDougall.com*, McDougall Research and Education Foundation, https://www.drmcdougall.com/health/education/health-science/common-health-problems/colitis-severe/
21. Kerr, Michael, "Nutritional Deficiencies and Crohn's Disease," *Healthline*, August 2018.
22. "The Dirty Secret of Government Drinking Water Standards," Environmental Working Group, October 2019, https://www.ewg.org/tapwater/state-of-american-drinking-water.php.
23. Ibid.
24. Mishra, Lakshmi-Chandra et al., "Scientific Basis for the Therapeutic Use of Withania somnifera (Ashwagandha): A Review," *Alternative Medicine Review*, 2000, vol. 5(4):334-46.
25. Khayyal, MT et al., "Mechanisms involved in the gastro-protective effect of STW 5 (Iberogast) and its components against ulcers and rebound acidity," *Phytomedicine*, 2006, 13(5):56-66.
26. S-M Elsas et al., "Passiflora incarnata L. (Passionflower) extracts elicit GABA currents in hippocampal neurons in vitro, and show anxiogenic and anticonvulsant effects in vivo, varying with extraction method," *Phytomedicine*, 2010, vol. 17(12):940-9.
27. Triantafyllidi, Aikaterini et al., "Herbal and plant therapy in patients with inflammatory bowel disease," *Annals of gastroenterology*, 2015, vol. 28(2):210-220.
28. "Boswellia serrata. Monograph." *Alternative Medicine Review*, 2008, vol. 13(2):165-7.
29. Hartmann, Renata Minuzzo et al., "Boswellia serrata has beneficial anti-inflammatory and antioxidant properties in a model of experimental colitis," *Phytotherapy Research*, 2014, vol. 28(9):1392-8.
30. Singla, Vikas et al., "Induction with NCB-02 (curcumin) enema for mild-to-moderate distal ulcerative colitis - a randomized, placebo-controlled, pilot study," *Journal of Crohn's & Colitis*, 2014, vol. 8(3):208-14.
31. Jurenka, Julie S., "Anti-inflammatory Properties of Curcumin, a Major Constituent of Curcuma longa: A Review of Preclinical and Clinical Research," *Alternative Medicine Review*, 2009, vol. 14(2):141-53.

32. Chainani-Wu, Nita, "Safety and anti-inflammatory activity of curcumin: a component of tumeric (Curcuma longa)," *Journal of Alternative and Complementary Medicine*, 2003, vol. 9(1):161-8.

33. Sareen, Rashmi et al., "Curcumin: a boon to colonic diseases," *Current Drug Targets*, 2013, vol. 14(10):1210-8.

34. Bright, John J., "Curcumin and autoimmune disease," *Advances in Experimental Medicine and Biology*, 2007, vol. 595:425-51.

35. Chandran, Binu, and Ajay Goel, "A randomized, pilot study to assess the efficacy and safety of curcumin in patients with active rheumatoid arthritis," *Phytotherapy Research*, 2012, vol. 26(11):1719-25.

36. Asakura H. and T. Kitahora, "Antioxidants in Inflammatory Bowel Disease, Ulcerative Colitis, and Crohn Disease," *Bioactive Food as Dietary Interventions for Liver and Gastrointestinal Disease*, Academic Press, 2013, pp. 37-53.

37. Langmead, L. et al., "Antioxidant effects of herbal therapies used by patients with inflammatory bowel disease: an in vitro study," *Alimentary Pharmacology & Therapeutics*, 2002, vol. 16:197-205.

38. Hawrelak, Jason A. and Stephen P. Myers, "Effects of Two Natural Medicine Formulations on Irritable Bowel Syndrome Symptoms: A Pilot Study," *The Journal of Alternative and Complementary Medicine*, 2010, vol. 16(10):1065-71.

39. Takhshid, Mohammad et al., "The healing effect of licorice extract in acetic acid-induced ulcerative colitis in rat model," *Comparative Clinical Pathology*, December 2012, vol. 21:1139-44.

40. Raveendra, Kadur Ramamurthy et al., "An Extract of Glycyrrhiza glabra (GutGard) Alleviates Symptoms of Functional Dyspepsia: A Randomized, Double-Blind, Placebo-Controlled Study," *Evidence-based Complementary and Alternative Medicine*, vol. 2012(2012):216970.

41. Dehpour, A.R. et al., "Antiulcer activities of liquorice and its derivatives in experimental gastric lesion induced by ibuprofen in rats," *International Journal of Pharmaceutics*, June 1995, vol. 119(2):133-8.

42. M Bortolotti and S Porta, "Effect of red pepper on symptoms of irritable bowel syndrome: preliminary study," *Digestive Diseases and Sciences*, 2011, vol. 56(11):3288-95.

43. Zmora, Niv et al., "Personalized Gut Mucosal Colonization Resistance to Empiric Probiotics Is Associated with Unique Host and Microbiome Features," *Cell*, September 2018, vol. 174(6):1388-1405.

44. Schink, M et al., "Microbial Patterns in Patients with Histamine Intolerance," *Journal of Physiology and Pharmacology*, 2018, vol. 69(4):579-93.

45. Suez, Jotham et al., "Post-Antibiotic Gut Mucosal Microbiome Reconstitution Is Impaired by Probiotics and Improved by Autologous FMT," *Cell*, September 2018, vol. 174(6):1406-23.

46. Mercola, Joseph, "An Interview with Dr. Natasha Campbell-McBride," Mercola.com, 12 May 2012.

47. Hou, Jason K et al., "Dietary intake and risk of developing inflammatory bowel disease: a systematic review of the literature," *American Journal of Gastroenterology*, April 2011, vol. 106(4):563-73.

48. Hubbard, Troy et al., "Dietary broccoli impacts microbial community structure and attenuates chemically induced colitis in mice in an Ah receptor dependent manner," *Journal of Functional Foods*, October 2017, vol. 37:685-98.

49. "Spinach, raw Nutrition Facts & Calories," Self.com, Conde Nast, https://nutritiondata.self.com/facts/vegetables-and-vegetable-products/2626/2.

50. Howell, Edward, *Enzyme Nutrition*, Penguin Putnam Inc., 1985, p. xi.

51. Hwang, In Guk et al., "Effects of Different Cooking Methods on the Antioxidant Properties of Red Pepper (Capsicum annuum L.)," *Preventive Nutrition and Food Science*, December 2012, vol. 17(4):286-92.

52. Klein, David, *Self Healing Colitis & Crohns*, Living Nutrition Publications, 26 October 2014, p. 42.

53. Russel, M G et al., "Modern life' in the epidemiology of inflammatory bowel disease: a case-control study with special emphasis on nutritional factors," *European Journal of Gastroenterology & Hepatology*, March 1998, vol. 10(3):243-9.

54. Wang, Li-Shu et al., "Dietary black raspberries modulate DNA methylation in dextran sodium sulfate (DSS)-induced ulcerative colitis." *Carcinogenesis*, December 2013, vol. 34(12):2842-50.

55. Yashiro, T et al., "Pterostilbene reduces colonic inflammation by suppressing dendritic cell activation and promoting regulatory T cell development," *The FASEB Journal,* September 2020, vol. 34:14810-9.

56. Topping, D L, and P M Clifton, "Short-chain fatty acids and human colonic function: roles of resistant starch and nonstarch polysaccharides," *Physiological Reviews*, July 2001, vol. 81(3):031-64.

57. Chiba, Mitsuro et al., "Recommendation of plant-based diets for inflammatory bowel disease," *Translational Pediatrics*, 2019, vol. 8(1):23-7.

58. Chiba, Mitsuro et al., "Plant-based diets in Crohn's disease," *The Permanente Journal*, Fall 2014, vol. 18(4):94.

59. Chiba, M et al., "Lifestyle-related disease in Crohn's disease: Relapse prevention by a semi-vegetarian diet," *World Journal of Gastroenterology*, May 2010, vol. 16(20):2484-95.

60. "Living with Crohn's Disease," The Crohn's and Colitis Foundation, October 2018, p. 17.

61. Chiba, Mitsuro et al., "Induction with Infliximab and a Plant-Based Diet as First-Line (IPF) Therapy for Crohn Disease: A Single-Group Trial." *The Permanente Journal*, October 2017, vol. 21:17-009.

62. Owczarek, Danuta et al., "Diet and nutritional factors in inflammatory bowel diseases." *World Journal of Gastroenterology*, January 2016, vol. 22(3):895-905.

63. Jantchou, Prévost et al., "Animal protein intake and risk of inflammatory bowel disease: The E3N prospective study." *The American Journal of Gastroenterology*, October 2010, vol. 105(10):2195-201.

64. Shoda, R, et al., "Epidemiologic Analysis of Crohn Disease in Japan: Increased Dietary Intake of N-6 Polyunsaturated Fatty Acids and Animal Protein Relates to the Increased Incidence of Crohn Disease in Japan," *The American Journal of Clinical Nutrition*, May 1996, vol. 63(5):741-5.

65. Tilg, H, and A Kaser, "Diet and relapsing ulcerative colitis: take off the meat?." *Gut*, October 2004, vol. 53(10):1399-401.

66. Levine, Morgan et al., "Low Protein Intake Is Associated with a Major Reduction in IGF-1, Cancer, and Overall Mortality in the 65 and Younger but Not Older Population," *Cell Metabolism*, March 2017, vol. 19(3):407-17.

67. Knox, E G. "Foods and diseases." *British Journal of Preventive & Social Medicine*, June 1977, vol. 31(2):71-80.

68. Kadoch MA. "Is the treatment of multiple sclerosis headed in the wrong direction? *Canadian Journal of Neurological Sciences*, May 2012, vol. 39(3):405.

69. Judaki, Arezo et al., "Evaluation of dairy allergy among ulcerative colitis patients." *Bioinformation*, November 2014, vol. 10(11):693-6.

70. Truelove, S C, "Ulcerative colitis provoked by milk." *British Medical Journal*, 1961, vol. 1(5220):154-60.

71. Sandefur, Kelsea et al., "Crohn's Disease Remission with a Plant-Based Diet: A Case Report," Nutrients vol. 11,6 1385. 20 Jun. 2019

72. "Egg, whole, raw, fresh Nutrition Facts & Calories," Self.com, Conde Nast, https://nutritiondata.self.com/facts/dairy-and-egg-products/111/2

73. Reif S, et al., "Pre-illness dietary factors in inflammatory bowel disease," *Gut*, 1997, vol. 40:754-60.

74. Andersson, H, "Fat-reduced diet in the symptomatic treatment of patients with ileopathy." *Nutrition and Metabolism*, 1974, vol. 17(2):102-11.

75. "Eggs Increase Risk for Heart Disease," Physicians Committee for Responsible Medicine, 1 July 2015.

76. Li, Yuehua et al, "Egg consumption and risk of cardiovascular diseases and diabetes: a meta-analysis," *Atherosclerosis*, August 2013, vol. 229(2):524-30.

77. Iscovich, J M et al, "Colon cancer in Argentina. I: Risk from intake of dietary items," *International Journal of Cancer*, July 1992, vol. 51(6):851-7.

78. McCance, RA et al., "Bone and vegetable broth," *Arch Dis Child*, August 1934, vol. 9(52):251-8.

79. Monro, J A et al., "The risk of lead contamination in bone broth diets," *Medical Hypotheses*, April 2013, vol. 80(4):389-90.

80. Heid, Markham, "Science Can't Explain Why Everyone is Drinking Bone Broth," *Time*, Time.com, 6 January 2016.

81. Shaw, MH and NE Flynn, "Amino Acid Content of Beef, Chicken, and Turkey Bone Broth," *Journal of Undergraduate Chemistry Research*, 2019, vol. 18(4):15-7.

82. Heyland, Daren et al., "A Randomized Trial of Glutamine and Antioxidants in Critically Ill Patients,"

83. Matijašić, Mario et al., "Modulating Composition and Metabolic Activity of the Gut Microbiota in IBD Patients," *International Journal of Molecular Sciences*, 19 April 2016, vol. 17(4)578.

84. Satokari R., "High Intake of Sugar and the Balance between Pro- and Anti-Inflammatory Gut Bacteria," *Nutrients*, 2020, vol. 12(5):1348.

85. Manzel, Arndt et al., "Role of "Western diet" in inflammatory autoimmune diseases," *Current Allergy and Asthma Reports*, January 2014, vol. 14(1):404.

86. Festen, Eleonora A M et al., "A meta-analysis of genome-wide association scans identifies IL18RAP, PTPN2, TAGAP, and PUS10 as shared risk loci for Crohn's disease and celiac disease," *PLoS Genetics*, January 2011, vol. 7(1):e1001283.

87. Herfarth, Hans H et al., "Prevalence of a gluten-free diet and improvement of clinical symptoms in patients with inflammatory bowel diseases," *Inflammatory Bowel Diseases,* July 2014, vol. 20(7):1194-7.

88. Makharia, Archita et al., "The Overlap between Irritable Bowel Syndrome and Non-Celiac Gluten Sensitivity: A Clinical Dilemma." *Nutrients*, 10 December 2015, vol. 7(12):10417-26.

89. Hallert, Claes et al., "Increasing fecal butyrate in ulcerative colitis patients by diet: controlled pilot study." *Inflammatory Bowel Diseases*, March 2003, vol. 9(2):116-21.

90. Abdo, Joe et al., "Interplay of Immunity and Vitamin D: Interactions and Implications with Current IBD Therapy," *Current Medicinal Chemistry*, 2017, vol. 24(9):852-867.

91. Rogler, Gerhard et al., "The Search for Causative Environmental Factors in Inflammatory Bowel Disease," *Digestive Diseases*, 22 August 2016, vol. 34(1):48-55.

92. Lock, S., "U.S. fast food restaurants statistics & facts," Statista, 9 December 2020,

93. Gearhardt, Ashley N et al., "Preliminary validation of the Yale Food Addiction Scale." *Appetite*, 2009, vol. 52(2):430-6.

94. Schulte, Erica M et al., "Which foods may be addictive? The roles of processing, fat content, and glycemic load," PloS One, February 2015, vol. 10(2): e0117959.

95. Baik, Ja-Hyun, "Dopamine signaling in food addiction: role of dopamine D2 receptors," *BMB Reports*, 2013, vol. 46(11):519-26.

96. Blum, Kenneth et al., "Dopamine and glucose, obesity, and reward deficiency syndrome," *Frontiers in Psychology*, September 2014, vol. 5:919.

97. Mayer, Emeran A, "Gut feelings: the emerging biology of gut-brain communication," *Nature Reviews Neuroscience*, July 2011, vol. 12(8):453-66.

98. Breit, Sigrid et al., "Vagus Nerve as Modulator of the Brain-Gut Axis in Psychiatric and Inflammatory Disorders," *Frontiers in Psychiatry*, March 2018, vol. 9:44.

99. Pellissier, Sonia et al., "Relationship between vagal tone, cortisol, TNF-alpha, epinephrine and negative affects in Crohn's disease and irritable bowel syndrome." *PloS One*, September 2014, vol. 9(9):e105328.
100. Clarke, Gerard et al., "Minireview: Gut microbiota: the neglected endocrine organ," *Molecular Endocrinology*, 2014, vol. 28(8):1221-38.
101. Yano, Jessica M et al., "Indigenous bacteria from the gut microbiota regulate host serotonin biosynthesis," *Cell*, 2015, vol. 161(2):264-76.
102. Mazzoli, Roberto, and Enrica Pessione, "The Neuro-endocrinological Role of Microbial Glutamate and GABA Signaling," *Frontiers in Microbiology*, November 2016, vol. 7:1934.
103. Wurtman, RJ, "Dietary Treatments That Affect Brain Neurotransmitters," *Annals of the New York Academy of Sciences*, 1987, vol. 499:179-190.
104. Moshfegh, Alanna et al., *What We Eat in America*, NHANES 2001-2002: Usual Nutrient Intakes from Food Compared to Dietary Reference Intakes, 2005, U.S. Department of Agriculture, Agricultural Research Service.
105. Dilzer, Allison et al., "The Family of Dietary Fibers," *Nutrition Today*, May/June 2013, vol. 48(3):108-18.
106. Hou, Jason K et al., "Dietary intake and risk of developing inflammatory bowel disease: a systematic review of the literature," *The American Journal of Gastroenterology*, vol. 106(4):563-73.
107. Brotherton, Carol et al., "Avoidance of Fiber Is Associated With Greater Risk of Crohn's Disease Flare in a 6-Month Period," *Clinical Gastroenterology and Hepatology*, August 2016, vol. 14(8):1130-6.
108. Chiba, Mitsuro et al., "High amount of dietary fiber not harmful but favorable for Crohn disease," *The Permanente Journal*, 2015, vol. 19(1):58-61.
109. Boekema, P J et al., "Coffee and gastrointestinal function: facts and fiction. A review," *Scandinavian Journal of Gastroenterology Supplement*, 1999, vol. 230:35-9.
110. Swanson, Garth R et al., "Pattern of alcohol consumption and its effect on gastrointestinal symptoms in inflammatory bowel disease," *Alcohol*, 2010, vol. 44(3): 223-8.
111. Magee, Elizabeth A et al. "Associations between diet and disease activity in ulcerative colitis patients using a novel method of data analysis." *Nutrition Journal*, 10 February 2005, vol. 4 7.
112. Jowett, SL et al., "Influence of dietary factors on the clinical course of ulcerative colitis: a prospective cohort study" *Gut*, 2004, vol. 53:1479-84.
113. Ahrens, S et al., "Almond (Prunus dulcis L.) Protein Quality," *Plant Foods for Human Nutrition*, 2005, vol. 60:123-8.
114. Neil Osterweil, "The Benefits of Protein," *WebMD*.
115. McDougall, John, "Plant foods have a complete amino acid composition," *Circulation*, June 2002, vol. 105(25):e197.
116. Levine, Morgan et al., "Low protein intake is associated with a major reduction in IGF-1, cancer, and overall mortality in the 65 and younger but not older population," *Cell Metabolism*, 2014, vol. 19(3):407-17.

117. Millward, D. Joe, "Identifying recommended dietary allowances for protein and amino acids: a critique of the 2007 WHO/FAO/UNU report," *The British Journal of Nutrition*, 2012, vol. 108(2):S3-21.

118. Institute of Medicine, *Dietary Reference Intakes: The Essential Guide to Nutrient Requirements*, Washington, DC: The National Academies Press, 2006, pp. 144-6.

119. Delimaris, Ioannis, "Adverse Effects Associated with Protein Intake above the Recommended Dietary Allowance for Adults," *ISRN Nutrition*, July 2013, vol. 2013.

120. InterAct Consortium et al., "Association between dietary meat consumption and incident type 2 diabetes: the EPIC-InterAct study." *Diabetologia*, 2013, vol. 56(1):47-59.

121. Tharrey, Marion et al., "Patterns of plant and animal protein intake are strongly associated with cardiovascular mortality: the Adventist Health Study-2 cohort," *International Journal of Epidemiology*, October 2018, vol. 47(5):1603-12.

122. Amy Joy Lanou, "Should dairy be recommended as part of a healthy vegetarian diet? Counterpoint," *The American Journal of Clinical Nutrition*, May 2009, vol. 89(5):1638S-42S.

123. Feskanich, D et al., "Milk, dietary calcium, and bone fractures in women: a 12-year prospective study," *American Journal of Public Health*, 1997, vol. 87(6): 992-7. see also Michaëlsson, Karl et al., "Dietary calcium and vitamin D intake in relation to osteoporotic fracture risk," *Bone*, vol. 32(6):694-703.

124. Adams, Kelly M et al., "Nutrition education in U.S. medical schools: latest update of a national survey," *Academic Medicine: Journal of the Association of American Medical Colleges*, 2010, vol. 85(9):1537-42.

125. Parker, Whadi-ah et al., "They think they know but do they? Misalignment of perceptions of lifestyle modification knowledge among health professionals," *Public Health Nutrition*, August 2009, vol. 14(8):1429-38.

126. Kushner, R F, "Barriers to providing nutrition counseling by physicians: a survey of primary care practitioners," *Preventive Medicine*, 1995, vol. 24(6):546-52.

127. "Physicians and pharmacy sales reps indicted for kickback conspiracy in which doctors allegedly received money in exchange for writing unnecessary prescriptions of Nuedexta," Department of Justice, U.S. Attorney's Office, Northern District of Ohio, 26 September 2019.

128. Mikulic, Matej, "U.S. pharmaceutical industry - statistics & facts," Statista.com, 5 November 2020, https://www.statista.com/topics/1719/pharmaceutical-industry/.

129. Neel, Joel, "Medical Schools and Drug Firm Dollars," NPR.org, 9 June 2005, https://www.npr.org/templates/story/story.php?storyId=4696316.

130. Howley, Elaine, "Do Drug Company Payments to Doctors Influence Which Drugs They Prescribe?" U.S. News, 31 August 2018, https://

health.usnews.com/health-care/patient-advice/articles/2018-08-31/do-drug-company-payments-to-doctors-influence-which-drugs-they-prescribe.
131. "Client Profile: Pharmaceutical Research & Manufacturers of America," Center for Responsive Politics, 2019, https://www.opensecrets.org/federal-lobbying/clients/summary?cycle=2019&id=D000000504.
132. Popkin, Barry, "Global nutrition dynamics: the world is shifting rapidly toward a diet linked with noncommunicable diseases," *The American Journal of Clinical Nutrition*, August 2006, vol. 84(2):289-98.
133. Chiba, Mitsuro et al., "Westernized Diet is the Most Ubiquitous Environmental Factor in Inflammatory Bowel Disease." *The Permanente Journal*, 2019, vol. 23:18-107.
134. Brown, Amy C et al., "Existing dietary guidelines for Crohn's disease and ulcerative colitis," *Expert Review of Gastroenterology & Hepatology*, 2011, vol. 5(3):411-25.
135. Rogler, Gerhard et al., "The Search for Causative Environmental Factors in Inflammatory Bowel Disease," *Digestive Diseases*, 2016, vol. 34(1):48-55.
136. Kimura, Yoshitaka et al., "Evaluation of the effects of mastication and swallowing on gastric motility using electrogastrography," *Journal of Medical Investigation*, 2006, vol. 53:229-37.
137. Hollis, James H, "The effect of mastication on food intake, satiety and body weight," *Physiology & Behavior*, 2018, vol. 193(B):242-5.
138. Cassady, Bridget A et al., "Mastication of almonds: effects of lipid bioaccessibility, appetite, and hormone response," *The American Journal of Clinical Nutrition*, March 2009, vol. 89(3):794–800.
139. Kumamoto, Carol A, "Inflammation and gastrointestinal Candida colonization," *Current Opinion in Microbiologyl*, 2011, vol. 14(4):386-91.

Printed in Great Britain
by Amazon

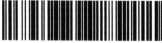